Nestlé Nutrition Institute Workshop Series

Vol. 78

International Nutrition: Achieving Millennium Goals and Beyond

Editors

Robert E. Black Baltimore, MD, USA
Atul Singhal London, UK
Ricardo Uauy Santiago, Chile

KARGER

Nestlé
Nutrition Institute

Nestec Ltd., 55 Avenue Nestlé, CH–1800 Vevey (Switzerland)
S. Karger AG, P.O. Box, CH–4009 Basel (Switzerland) www.karger.com

Library of Congress Cataloging-in-Publication Data

Nestlé Nutrition Workshop (78th : 2013 : Muscat, Oman), author.
  International nutrition : achieving millennium goals and beyond / editors,
Robert E. Black, Atul Singhal, Ricardo Uauy.
    p. ; cm. -- (Nestlé Nutrition Institute workshop series, ISSN
1664-2147 ; vol. 78)
  Includes bibliographical references and index.
  ISBN 978-3-318-02530-9 (hard cover : alk. paper) -- ISBN 978-3-318-02531-6
(e-ISBN)
  I. Black, Robert E., editor of compilation. II. Singhal, Atul, editor of
compilation. III. Uauy, Ricardo, editor of compilation. IV. Nestlé Nutrition
Institute, issuing body. V. Title. VI. Series: Nestlé Nutrition Institute
workshop series ; v. 78. 1664-2147
  [DNLM: 1. Child Nutritional Physiological Phenomena--Congresses. 2.
Child Welfare--Congresses. 3. Internationality--Congresses. 4. Nutritional
Requirements--Congresses. 5. World Health--Congresses. W1 NE228D v.78 2014
/ WS 130]
  RJ102
  362.19892--dc23
                                                      2013043551

Printed on acid-free and non-aging paper
ISBN 978–3–318–02530–9
e-ISBN 978–3–318–02531–6
ISSN 1664–2147
e-ISSN 1664–2155

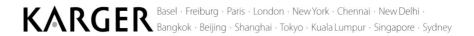

KARGER Basel · Freiburg · Paris · London · New York · Chennai · New Delhi · Bangkok · Beijing · Shanghai · Tokyo · Kuala Lumpur · Singapore · Sydney

Contents

For more information on related publications, please consult the NNI website: www.nestlenutrition–institute.org

Preface

The UN Millennium Development Goals Report 2012 says: 'Despite clear evidence of the disastrous consequences of childhood nutritional deprivation in the short and long terms, nutritional health remains a low priority. It is time for nutrition to be placed higher on the development agenda.' The 78th Nestlé Nutrition Institute Workshop, which took place in Oman in March 2013, focused on improving the nutrition and health of young women and children.

The first session was dedicated to the analysis of world nutrition situation in achieving Millennium Development Goal (MDG) 1. The presentations were designed in a way to cover the global distribution of malnutrition and micronutrient deficiencies in world population of young women and infants and disease burden related to it. A separate topic focused on the implementation of strategies and policies that can reduce infant and maternal morbidity and mortality during the first 1,000 days.

The second session of the workshop covered the interventions that have been and could be deployed to help achieve the MDGs, particularly the nutrition component of MDG 1 and MDGs 4 and 5 on reducing child and maternal mortality. With less than 3 years remaining before the MDG target date of 2015, there is increasing commitment and urgency for scaling up all proven interventions that will have the needed impact. The presentations in this session were designed to review the evidence on ways to achieve the MDGs and the potential contributions of nutrition-specific and disease control interventions, as well as the possible role of sectors other than health. Two presentations considered broadly the maternal and child interventions, including those that are being implemented but could be brought to greater scale and those that could be implemented now given current knowledge on their effects. Two presentations reviewed the issues regarding maternal undernutrition, fetal growth restriction and gain in length and weight in childhood and implications for stunting and adult noncommunicable diseases. The fifth presentation was selected to explore the possible contributions of agriculture to nutrition and the MDGs. It is expected that reduction of poverty will help achievement of all of the MDGs, but enhanced agriculture may have particular contributions to make for the MDGs that are the focus in this workshop.

The final session of the workshop, at first glance, appeared out of step with the previous two sessions and the overall theme of the meeting. However, while meeting the MDGs is the most important priority for many lower-income countries (as highlighted by earlier speakers), many countries in transition face a 'double burden' of disease, with noncommunicable disease fast becoming the predominant health issue facing rich and poor populations alike. The aim of this last session therefore was to look into the future and highlight the problems of obesity, cardiovascular disease and atopic disease which emerging countries will face within the next 20 years.

The four presentations in the last session covered the causes and consequences of noncommunicable disease in both the developing and developed world, reviewed the latest scientific evidence for underlying mechanisms, and discussed the implications for public health and policy makers. Speakers highlighted the impact of early feeding practices (in fetal life, early infancy and early childhood) on programming the risk of noncommunicable disease, as well as the role of nutrition and other environmental factors throughout the life course in predisposing to chronic disease. As always, presentations were followed by lively discussion particularly on the more controversial scientific hypotheses such as the impact of infant growth on the risk of later obesity and cardiovascular disease, and emerging data on the importance of the microbiome in the development of atopic eczema and other allergic conditions. Although more research is clearly needed, the message was clear – lessons need to be learnt from both the developed and developing world in order to stem the current global epidemic of noncommunicable disease.

On behalf of all participants, we are particularly indebted to Prof. Ferdinand Haschke – Head of Nestlé Nutrition Institute, and his team for providing this fantastic opportunity for discussion and learning. Thank you.

Robert E. Black
Atul Singhal
Ricardo Uauy

Foreword

The Nestlé Nutrition Institute has previously organized several workshops in the field of public health and nutrition [1–3]. This time, for the 78th Nestlé Nutrition Institute Workshop in Oman, the theme 'International Nutrition – Achieving Millennium Goals and Beyond' was chosen. During the workshop, international target setting was discussed as we looked into how it has been used to influence health outcomes in two highly important segments of the world population – young women and their children. The workshop was the first Nestlé Nutrition Institute event with global broadcasting; it allowed us to share this fantastic program with thousands of scientists around the world.

The world nutrition situation was analyzed, including evidence how country-level action can influence nutrition, in particular agricultural and nutritional interventions. We learned about the strong influence global distribution of resources has on the burden of disease: infant feeding practices in 20 developing countries are associated with improved growth and lower burden of disease. Despite all efforts to support breastfeeding, the question was addressed why only 30–40% of infants are exclusively breastfed until 6 months of age and what can be done to improve the situation. As far as the infant food industry is concerned, there is a need to work with governmental agencies and NGOs and to follow and respect the country-specific interpretation of the WHO code on marketing of breast milk substitutes.

Evidence on interventions and field studies indicated that maternal undernutrition and micronutrient deficiencies are strongly related to low birthweight. Providing women of reproductive age with adequate nutrition is key for successful pregnancy outcome and breastfeeding. Monitoring growth of infants and children to prevent or correct micronutrient deficiencies can have a lifelong effect: iron deficiency anemia with its negative effect on brain function was addressed as an example.

Nutrition during the fetal and postnatal periods was also discussed due to the rising recognition of its value as a means of preventing noncommunicable diseases such as obesity and related complications – diabetes, cardiovascular diseases and stroke. Interventions in developing and developed countries must address maternal obesity [4] as well as fetal and postnatal nutrition – the critical period of the first 1,000 days. Another important topic was prevention of allergic disease and atopic dermatitis through early nutritional intervention. It can now be concluded that such a strategy may help reduce the burden of diseases such as chronic lung disease.

We would like to thank the three chairmen for putting the program together: Prof. Robert E. Black, Prof. Ricardo Uauy, and Prof. Atul Singhal.

We would also like to thank the speakers, moderators and scientific experts in the audience, who have contributed to the workshop content and professional discussions.

Finally, we thank George Salem, Anwar Hanan and their teams from Nestlé Nutrition Middle East for their logistic support.

References

1 Black R, Michaelsen KF (eds): Public Health Issues in Infant and Child Nutrition. Nestlé Nutr Workshop Ser. Vevey, Nestec, 2000, vol 48, view publication.
2 Bhatia J, Bhutta ZA, Kalhan SC (eds): Maternal and Child Nutrition: The First 1000 Days. Nestlé Nutr Workshop Ser. Vevey, Nestec/Basel, Karger, 2013, vol 74.
3 Drewnowski A, Rolls BJ (eds): Obesity Treatment and Prevention: New Directions. Nestlé Nutr Workshop Ser. Vevey, Nestec/Basel, Karger, 2012, vol 73.
4 Haschke F: Evaluation of growth and early infant feeding: a challenge for scientists, industry and regulatory bodies; in Shamir R, Turck D, Phillip M (eds): Nutrition and Growth. World Rev Nutr Diet. Basel, Karger, 2013, vol 106, pp 33–38.

Dr. Natalia Wagemans, MD, PhD
Global Medical Advisor
Nestlé Nutrition Institute
Vevey, Switzerland

Prof. Ferdinand Haschke, MD, PhD
Chairman
Nestlé Nutrition Institute
Vevey, Switzerland

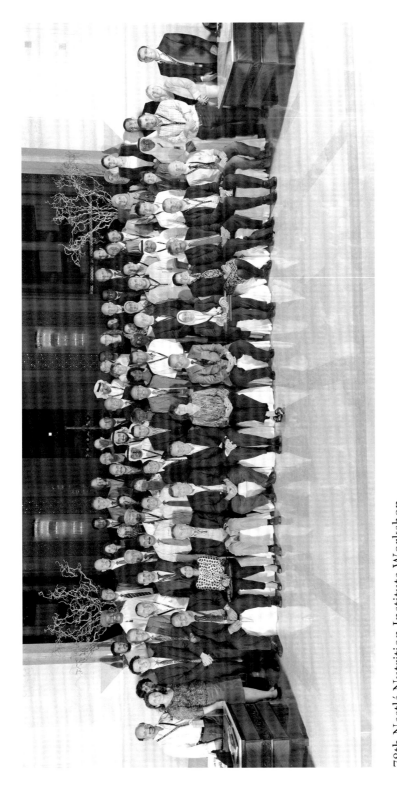

78th Nestlé Nutrition Institute Workshop
Muscat, March 20–22, 2013

Contributors

Chairpersons & Speakers

Prof. Linda S. Adair
Carolina Population Center
UNC Chapel Hill
Campus Box 8140
123 West Franklin St.
Chapel Hill, NC 27516-2524
USA
E-Mail linda_adair@unc.edu

Prof. Zulfiqar A. Bhutta
Aga Khan University
Stadium Road
PO Box 3500
Karachi 74800
Pakistan
E-Mail zulfiqar.bhutta@aku.edu

Prof. Robert E. Black
Johns Hopkins Bloomberg School of
Public Health
Department of International Health
615 N. Wolfe Street, Room E-8527
Baltimore, MD 21205
USA
E-Mail rblack@jhsph.edu

Prof. Parul Christian
Johns Hopkins Bloomberg School of
Public Health
Department of International Health
Center for Human Nutrition
615 N. Wolfe Street
Room 2541
Baltimore, MD 21205
USA
E-Mail pchristi@jhsph.edu

Prof. Andrew Dorward
Centre for Development, Environment
and Policy
School of Oriental and Africa Studies
(SOAS)
University of London
36 Gordon Square
London WC1H 0PD
UK
E-Mail Andrew.Dorward@soas.ac.uk

Prof. Ralf G. Heine
Department of Gastroenterology &
Clinical Nutrition
Department of Allergy & Immunology
Royal Children's Hospital Melbourne
Murdoch Children's Research Institute
University of Melbourne
Flemington Road
Parkville, VIC 3052
Australia
E-Mail ralf.heine@rch.org.au

Prof. Jorge Jiménez
Departamento de Salud Pública
Facultad de Medicina PUC
Marcoleta 434
Santiago de Chile
Chile
E-Mail jjimenez@med.puc.cl

Prof. Anoop Misra
Fortis-C-DOC Centre
C6/57 (ground floor)
Safdarjang Development Area
New Delhi 16
India
E-Mail anoopmisra@gmail.com

Prof. Lynnette M. Neufeld
Director, Monitoring, Learning and
Research
Global Alliance for Improved Nutrition
PO Box 55
1211 Geneva 20
Switzerland
E-Mail lneufeld@gainhealth.org

Prof. Andrew M. Prentice
MRC International Nutrition Group
Nutrition & Public Health Intervention
Research Unit
London School of Hygiene & Tropical
Medicine
Keppel Street
London WC1E 7HT
UK
E-Mail andrew.prentice@lshtm.ac.uk

Prof. Usha Ramakrishnan
Emory University
1519 Clifton Road NE
Atlanta, GA 30322
USA
E-Mail uramakr@sph.emory.edu

Prof. Atul Singhal
UCL Institute of Child Health
30 Guilford Street
London WC1N 1EH
UK
E-Mail a.singhal@ucl.ac.uk

Prof. Ricardo Uauy
INTA Universidad de Chile
Macul 5540
Santiago 11
Chile
E-Mail druauy@gmail.com

Prof. Benjamin O. Yarnoff
RTI International
3040 E. Cornwallis Road
Research Triangle Park, NC 27709
USA
E-Mail byarnoff@rti.org

Participants

Ayman AbdelRahim/Bahrain
Mohamed AlRefaei/Bahrain
Hasan Isa/Bahrain
Saheera Saleh/Bahrain
Christiane Leite/Brazil
Hugo Ribeiro Junior/Brazil
Mahmoud Alzalabany/Egypt
Mohamed Shaltout/Egypt
Simich Rita/Hungary
Arunkumar Desai/India
Shrawan Kumar/India
Jameela Kunjachan/India
Archisman Mohapatra/India
Sunil Kumar Nag/India
Ray Basrowi/Indonesia
Badriul Hegar/Indonesia
Wenny Lazdya Taifur/Indonesia
Mario De Curtis/Italy
Bashar AlKhasawneh/Jordan
Ali Almatti/Jordan
Samir Faouri/Jordan
Furat Kreishan/Jordan
Mohammad Rawashdeh/Jordan
Hussein Wahbeh/Jordan
Eiman Alenaizi/Kuwait
Hanan Ben Nekhi/Kuwait
Raafat Raad/Kuwait
Fadi Chamseddine/Lebanon
Mariam El Abdallah El Rajab/Lebanon
Bernard Gerbaka/Lebanon
Bassam Ghanem/Lebanon
Patricia Hoyek/Lebanon
Tahera Al Lawati/Oman
Tawfiq Al-Lawati/Oman
Salim Al Maskary/Oman
Mariam Al Waili/Oman
Huda Al Zidi/Oman
Ezzat Abdel Aziz/Oman
Mohey Hasanein/Oman
Salah Salem/Oman
Yaser Wali/Oman
Huma Fahim/Pakistan
Kadil Jr Sinolinding/Philippines
Grace Uy/Philippines
Mohamed Al Jamal/Qatar
Mohamed Kayyali/Qatar
Ahmed Masoud/Qatar
Fahmi Nasser/Qatar
Elena Lukushkina/Russia
Nayel Abdaly/Saudi Arabia
Mohammed Al Amrani/Saudi Arabia

Mohammed Al Tamran/Saudi Arabia
Hatem Alhani/Saudi Arabia
Khalid Almanee/Saudi Arabia
Ali Alshamrani/Saudi Arabia
Saeed Dolgum/Saudi Arabia
Omar Saadah/Saudi Arabia
Harbi Shawoosh/Saudi Arabia
Marco Turini/Singapore
Tengku Marina Badlishah/Switzerland
Denis Barclay/Switzerland

Yannick Evrard/Switzerland
Mael Guillemot/Switzerland
Hanan Anwar/United Arab Emirates
Mohammad Cheikhali/United Arab Emirates
Mohammad Howidi/United Arab Emirates
Sherif Mosaad/United Arab Emirates
Mahmoud Tana/United Arab Emirates
Sameh Zakher/United Arab Emirates

Black RE, Singhal A, Uauy R (eds): International Nutrition: Achieving Millennium Goals and Beyond.
Nestlé Nutr Inst Workshop Ser, vol 78, pp 1–10, (DOI: 10.1159/000354927)
Nestec Ltd., Vevey/S. Karger AG., Basel, © 2014

Country-Level Action to Improve Nutrition and Health: A View from the Field

Jorge Jiménez

Pontificia Universidad Católica de Chile, Santiago de Chile, Chile

Abstract

Preference for mother and child social protection is a constant in public policies all around the world. Most of the basic strategies are known and have been described, proven on its efficacy and cost-effectiveness several times in different settings in the last 100 years. But from knowledge to action and from action to impact, there has been a variable and dramatic gap which can be mended with other policy tools. Beyond technical considerations, conviction, commitment and mystique are in my view and experience those critical factors. The other issue is close relation between academia, policy making, regular politics and public opinion. © 2014 Nestec Ltd., Vevey/S. Karger AG, Basel

Here, I recall personal experience and review mother and child health (MCH) policies in the last 50 or more years in Chile, the country I know best [1–3].

The first registered event on child health policy in Chile took place in 1912. Many interventions with progressive coverage were implemented during decades of improvement in health care policies. The early emphasis on nutrition is quite clear from the start.

With the consolidation of a National Health Service (NHS) in the 1950s, Chile established an MCH policy based on the typical pillars of action: antenatal care, professional attention of deliveries, family planning, nutrition programs, well baby clinics, immunizations, respiratory and gastrointestinal infection therapies and water and sanitation projects in poor communities.

The basic ideas were developed and tested by a group of socially sensitive academics from Universidad de Chile, who went to the community, studied the sociomedical conditions, proposed and essayed their interventions (1955–1960) and after having the conviction, 'took power' by accessing key posts in the NHS (1960–1965).

Impact was visible by the late 1970s, ironically during a period of military dictatorship, neoliberal reforms to the economy and deep recessions. The sociomedical model for child survival proved to be stronger than reality would have predicted.

Background to Child Survival Policy

Infant and child health policies have been present in public health for more than two centuries together with maternal health and fertility intervention models. Together with infectious disease control, they are the main highlights of public policy, social priority and political platforms in every country regardless of the level of their development.

Reviewing history in Western countries we find all sorts of initiatives that reveal a universal motivation to save children's lives. From charity to legislation with pro-poor and pro-children protection laws and governmental provisions; together with industry production of effective food for babies and global agencies maternal and child health policy formulations [4–6].

In my opinion, one of the best packaged policy formulations of child survival policy was GOBI, declared by UNICEF in the 1970s. G standing for growth and nutrition, O for oral rehydration in diarrheas, B for birth spacing and fertility regulation, and I for immunizations [7].

Later in the 21st century, one lucid conceptualization of infant and child survival awareness was the series of papers and policy convocations done by the Bellagio Group on Child Survival (2003) and published in *The Lancet*. In these publications of expert opinions, the main ideas were:
- Unacceptable high number of children are dying every year, 10 million
- Malnutrition is present in about 40% of cases
- We have cost-effective tools to prevent and treat the majority of negative conditions

We can see that the information has been there for a long time, many scholastic interpretations and theories have flourished, including the last one called Social Determinants of Health (UNICEF/Experts consultation 22–23 June 2012), but still too many children die at early stages of life with avoidable causes and the quality of life of these children is rather poor. This therefore is, as it always has been, a moral issue.

From Social Sensibility to Research, Action and Impact: The Case of Chile

Describing and reflecting on country-level experience is critical to correctly apply and establish solutions for survival and quality of life for children. Of course, there are many contextual conditions that restrict generalizations and simplistic attempts to teach or learn from others' experiences, and I will try to avoid that trap.

Between a National Conference on Infant Protection in 1912, headed by the President of the Republic, to the first explicit formulations of country policy documents in the 1960s and 1970s, several events occurred. Private charities appeared, public institutions were created, important research took place and several interventions were field tested by academics working in coordination with the health services network and planning centers. A chronological list is presented in table 1.

Formation and Influence of Leading Academics

Looking back and examining in more detail how things happened and which were the motivations for these developments, I found a group, not isolated but emblematic, that did things well, Prof. Meneghello's group. By mid-1950s, in the midst of creating the NHS with its ability to integrate different strengths from diverse sources, they established themselves as academics with a social mission.

Among other documents, they had a 'research manifesto' with some statements like: 'We shall put more interest in important than rare matters, in persons than in cases. As much interest in health as in disease, in prevention as in cure, in parents and families as in the child.'

In 1958, the main items in their research agenda, very much oriented to action, were the following, transcribed literally:
- Biodemographics of the district in charge
- Morbidity registration
- Evaluation of children's nutrition
- Evaluation of psychomotor development
- Longitudinal study of physical, biochemical and emotional states in different stages of development
- Useful research to define feeding models for children
- Evaluation of therapeutic norms in ambulatory care in its efficacy and cost
- Immunological studies to test the efficacy of vaccines in use
- In-depth analysis of sociodemographic, housing, cultural and environmental conditions of families

Table 1. Chronological list of developments, interventions and events related to health care in Chile

Time period	Institutional development, intervention, event	Infant mortality range, deaths per 1,000 LB
1900–1920	Goutte de Lait (1902) National Infant Protection Conference (1912)	300–247
1921–1940	Ministry of Health (1924) Mother and Child Health Law (1937) First National Council for Nutrition and Food (1937) First powdered milk factory in alliance with private industry and expansion of supplementary food programs (1937)	258–192
1941–1960	Agency for Infancy Protection (PROTINFA, 1942) NHS (1952) with integration of social security and medical and sanitary services Massive immunization and eradication of smallpox (1950–1954) Social Pediatrics Departments created by Universidad de Chile (1948–1954) First pilot interventions in community child health (1954–1960)	178–126
1961–1990	National Diarrhea Program is established (1964) Measles vaccine introduced in progressive universal coverage (1963) Universal access to – supplementary food programs (1965–1975) – second National Council for Nutrition (1974) – contraceptives and family planning services (1965) Midwife formation by Universidad de Chile reaches effective numbers (1970) Deliveries reach 98% professional care (1980) Water and sanitation reach 97 and 78% coverage Malnutrition rates fall from 37% of children under 6 years to 2.9% (2000) Average years of schooling for young women reaches 12 years	106–16
1991–2010	Second phase in child survival declared (1990) Universal access interventions established in – Consolidation of neonatal program – Expansion of vaccine program: HiB, MMR, 2nd dose of measles – National acute respiratory infections program – Congenital cardiac defects diagnosis and surgery Eradication of measles (1992) Fall in infant mortality rate due to pneumonia from 239 per 100,000 (1990) to 76 (2000) Health reform: Guarantee Program (2005) High-school and university students start massive protest for better education: demographic transition takes place	16–8

- Evaluation of the effect of sanitary education campaigns
- Execution of an effective antenatal control program and an obstetrical service that allows optimal and integral prenatal, newborn and postpartum care
- Comparative evaluation of present procedures in order to measure the performance of an MCH program and innovations suggested as experimental

One can see that this list of research and action should be presented as pertaining to the year 2013, and very few would discover that they are 55 years old and still valid.

I met these persons during my medical studies in the 1960s and was fascinated by their spirit, clearness of mind, commitment to do good and be part of a mystical project. They inspired people, inspired my own life.

At the beginning of 1960, a subgroup of more policy-motivated experts of these academics enrolled themselves in the NHS technical units via public opposition and started their escalation of programs in MCH strategies. With a high profile of conviction and consensus with other specialists and national politicians, their local models progressively became national. The country was living a time of social reform and search for ways to escape poverty and underdevelopment. In my international experience, perhaps the Finnish group of Pekka Pushka may parallel a similar access to political power for public health improvement purposes. The important lesson is: don't wait for the mountain to move towards you, go for it [pers. commun., 1998].

Continuing their career, these experts moved in the 1070s to the Pan American Health Organization (PAHO/WHO) and more or less repeated the same process with renowned success [8].

Impact of Policy

Results of infant mortality decline between 1950 through 2000 are shown in table 2.

Nutrition Policies over Time

As stated before, malnutrition of children is one of the most cited factors in infant mortality documents regarding diagnosis and strategies in the Chilean literature. The adoption of the private model of Goutte de Lait (milk drop) with fluid milk donation and later with well baby clinics was established in the country by pious ladies as a charity in 1903. In 1924, the Workers Insurance Institute (Caja de Seguro Obrero Obligatorio) rapidly adopted care for wives and children

Table 2. Infant mortality rate by selected causes, rates per 1,000 LB, Chile 1950–2000

	Year					
	1950	1960	1970	1980	1990	2000
LB number	208,092	287,063	251,231	247,013	307,522	261,993
Infant mortality rate	136.2	119.5	82.2	33.0	16.0	8.9
Neonatal mortality rate	50.4	34.6	31.7	16.7	8.5	5.6
Postneonatal mortality rate	85.8	84.9	50.5	16.3	7.5	3.3
Certain conditions originating in the perinatal period	38.7	47.8	17.5	12.9	5.5	3.4
Pneumonia and bronchopneumonia	44.4	31.0	19.5	4.2	2.4	0.7
Diarrhea and gastroenteritis of presumed infectious origin	29.0	16.0	15.2	2.0	0.24	0.0
Congenital malformations, deformations and chromosomal abnormalities	1.5	2.0	3.4	4.0	3.7	3.0
Selected infectious diseases: vaccination preventable, congenital syphilis and meningococcal infections	5.9	4.9	1.6	0.3	0.1	0.1

Author's analysis of data provided by the National Statistics Institute and the Ministry of Health, Chile.

of laborers ascribed to the scheme with expansions towards the end of the decade. The Mother and Child Law of 1937 was basically a pro-poor food and nutrition legislation with agreements between government, farmers producing milk and private industry putting technology for powdered and condensed milk production locally. Negotiations headed by the Minister of Health, a brilliant physician and inspired politician, took only a few months and the society adopted the strategy as its own.

By the mid-1940s, the difference between those protected by social insurance and the poor indigent families became evident, and a movement towards reforms headed by pediatricians and sensible politicians started in the country. Evidence was published and proclaimed by socially sensitive pediatricians with political connections.

The integration of different scattered services and social security medical units into an NHS became law in 1952 and progressively developed its algorithms for interventions mainly in MCH with a strong emphasis on nutrition programs.

The key set of interventions were the well baby control and included powdered milk donation, immunizations, basic therapy for infections (respiratory and intestinal) and maternal education.

In figure 1, it can be seen that there is a strong correlation between medical visits and the amount of milk distributed.

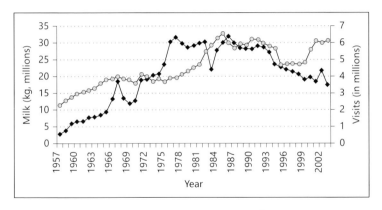

Fig. 1. Correlation between medical visits and the amount of milk distributed (1957–2003 MINSAL).

Table 3. Percentage of malnourished children under 6 years of age, Chile 1960–2000 [9]

Year	Total malnutrition	Mild	Moderate	Severe
1960	37.0	31.1	4.1	1.8
1970	19.3	15.8	2.5	1.0
1980	11.5	10.0	1.4	0.2
1990	8.0	7.7	0.2	0.1
2000	2.9	2.6	0.2	0.1

The impact of this nutrition policy, embedded into an integrated delivery of social services based on the Primary Health Care network of the Chilean NHS covering a high percentage of the territory and population was visible by the decade of 1970, and child malnutrition disappeared almost totally by the end of the century (table 3).

As we are now confronting the obesity epidemic, we may discuss the plausibility of these powdered milk donations linked with well baby care in the primary health care setting. The 'hook' is comparable to what now is called 'conditioned cash transfers' promoted by development agencies in child survival programs. But it is clear for me that the ensemble was a virtuous one.

Mortality Declines but Components Change: The Second Phase

By 1990, 40 years after the creation of the NHS, infant mortality had fallen to 16 per 1,000 live births (LB), a reduction of 88%. The main components were perinatal conditions with 5.5 per 1,000 LB (35%), congenital malformations with a rate of 3.7 (23%), and respiratory infections with 2.4 per 1,000 (16%). The neonatal component had surpassed the postneonatal fraction in a few years. This decline occurred in Chile in a period in which several recessions, hyperinflation and unemployment took place. In fact, the good evolution of infant and child survival proved to be independent of economic cycles. Nevertheless, towards 1990, the country was still only partly developed and had 40% of its population living under the poverty line, and faced a new challenge to its child health policy. Together with the restoration of democracy in 1990, the new government had to reinforce the social medicine and public health tradition of the country and express its commitment to improve equity in health.

Main interventions via specific programs were:
- Improved perinatal care via better technology and low birthweight prevention
- Treatment at primary health care of the acute respiratory infections, with innovative approaches
- Surgical correction of congenital heart disease
- Further expansion of the immunization program (measles second dose, HiB conjugate vaccine)

Results of the Second Phase Strategy

Infant mortality fell from 16 per 1,000 LB in 1990 to 8.9 in 2000. The biggest reductions were in: acute respiratory infections, from a rate of 2.4 to 0.66 per 1,000 LB; perinatal conditions, from 5.5 to 3.4 deaths per 1,000 LB, and congenital malformations, from 3.7 to 3.0 deaths per 1,000 LB (19% reduction; table 4). With the surgical program, mortality due to cardiac congenital conditions decreased from 1.24 to 0.82 per 1,000 LB (34% reduction). The total infant mortality rate of 8.9 had a totally changed composition, with almost two thirds (5.6) due to neonatal mortality and one third postneonatal (table 4). The total public health budget of Chile for 2000 was equivalent to USD 2.28 billion. The expenditure on these four innovative programs was USD 16.75 million, a minute fraction of the total. If we calculate that 285 additional children are surviving every year, each death averted costs near USD 58,771.

Lessons and Reflections

In my opinion, the main lessons behind this success story, from the public health point of view, were: (a) an integrated vision of health and life cycle with the environment, with a preference for health care in ambulatory and community settings;

Table 4. Infant and neonatal mortality by selected causes, 1990–2000 variation, Chile

Selected cause	Rate per 100,000 LB		Percent reduction
	1990	2000	1990–2000
Infant mortality due to pneumonia and bronchopneumonia	239.0	66.4	72.2
Infant mortality due to congenital cardiac disease	124.2	81.7	34.2
Neonatal mortality due to respiratory distress syndrome	64.4	33.2	48.4
Infant mortality	16,800	9,400	44
Neonatal mortality	8,900	5,900	33.7
Infant mortality due to congenital malformations	385.8	311.0	19.4

Author's analysis of data provided by the National Statistics Institute and the Ministry of Health, Chile.

(b) an integrated conception of health care and health organizations, in which every action is part of a holistic strategy; (c) a multidisciplinary health care team with several professions combining higher to lower skills with substitution of functions; (d) research and training in action through integration of public health services within university departments; (e) continuing evaluation of programs and instruments, and (f) permanent improvement of quality and reliability of epidemiological data, including medical certificate of cause of death and audit of infant deaths.

Integration is a key word and concept; it has to do with closeness between research and action, government and academia, public and private sectors; it is possible and necessary. If academics do not have power, they must look for it. The role of the private sector must be clearly defined and promoted beyond preconceived ideological positions in a pragmatic way.

The integrated conception of life and health is crucial; we always have to keep in mind that health is the consequence of multiple, especially social, factors and we must intervene on them from the societal level and by the provision of services. The link between health and nutrition is obvious.

The integration of care and different skills has proven to be critical in the expansion of health services. We are reinventing the wheel today with apparent innovative calls to build integrated services over the successful vertical programs such as HIV and tuberculosis (some people have very little memory).

Institutional arrangements to promote space for consensus are critical. National Councils or Boards such as the ones being used in several countries for vaccine and immunization policy are a good example of how different players can develop their part in a productive way.

Gender issue is also relevant for the construction of policy and creation of effective human resource networks. The role of women, again nothing new, is more than relevant in this objective.

The result of the child survival revolution takes us to a different and even more challenging stage: the demographic transition and the quality of life in early development. This is the situation we are facing today in Chile, with millions of teenagers demanding better education and training.

In summary, Chile shows a particular blend of applied research, close link between policy making and academia, field testing in local conditions, and above all, strong commitment with social policies for the society as a whole.

Disclosure Statement

The author received partial support for policy analysis in maternal and child health from Nestle Chile.

References

1 Jimenez J, Romero M: Reducing infant mortality in Chile, success in two phases. Health Affairs 2007;26:458–465.

2 Jimenez J: Angelitos salvados. Santiago, Uqbar Editores, 2009.

3 Jimenez J: Construir políticas infantiles desde la ciencia y la mística. Rev Chil Pediatr 2010; 81:295–299.

4 Claeson M, Bos ER, Mawji T, Pathmanathan I: Reducing child mortality in India in the new millennium. Bull World Health Organ 2000;78:1192–1199.

5 Clemens M: Africa's child health miracle: the biggest, best story in development. http://blogs.cgdev.org/globaldevelopment/2012/05/africas-child-health-miracle-the-biggest-best-story-in-development.php.

6 Yarrow AL: History of US Children's Policy 1900–Present. Washington, First Focus, 2009.

7 http://www.unicef.org/sowc96/1980s.htm.

8 Jimenez de la Jara J: Abraham Horwitz (1910–2000): a leading man of Pan American Public Health (in Spanish). Rev Med Chil 2003;131:929–934.

9 Monckeberg F: Prevention of malnutrition in Chile, experience lived by an actor and spectator. Rev Chil Nutr 2003;30(suppl 1):160–176.

Black RE, Singhal A, Uauy R (eds): International Nutrition: Achieving Millennium Goals and Beyond.
Nestlé Nutr Inst Workshop Ser, vol 78, pp 11–19, (DOI: 10.1159/000354930)
Nestec Ltd., Vevey/S. Karger AG., Basel, © 2014

Global, Regional and Country Trends in Underweight and Stunting as Indicators of Nutrition and Health of Populations

L.M. Neufeld · S.J.M. Osendarp

Micronutrient Initiative, Ottawa, ON, Canada

Abstract

Stunting and wasting provide indicators of different nutritional deficiency problems, the causes of which are well established. Underweight based on weight-for-age cannot distinguish between these two and is therefore not useful to target programs and has limited value for tracking progress. Stunting reduces later school attainment and income as adults and increases the risk of obesity and noncommunicable diseases in later life. Globally, the estimated number of stunted children is decreasing, but is not on track to meet the goal of 100 million by 2025 (165 million), and there has been little change in the number of children suffering from wasting since 2004. Stunting and wasting provide excellent indicators of inequity. For example, from 1990 to 2010, the number of stunted children in Asia declined from 188.7 to 98.4 million, while in sub-Saharan Africa there was essentially no change in prevalence, and the number of stunted children increased from 45.7 to 55.8 million. Recent global development movements are recognizing the need for robust measures of trends in nutritional status of children, particularly during the critical first years of life. Such measures are needed to track progress and improve accountability, and should be aspirational to mobilize sufficient investment in nutrition.

Undernutrition as an Indicator of the Nutrition and Health of Populations

Healthy growth occurs as a result of adequate dietary intake, care-giving, including feeding practices, and a low burden of infectious disease [1]. Insufficient food intake to meet protein and energy needs leads to acute malnutrition (wasting, low weight-for-height), the severity of which will depend on the duration and size of the deficit. Wasting is usually associated with chronic or acute periods of food insecurity and exacerbated by infectious disease [2]. Linear growth faltering or stunting (low height-for-age) is the result of insufficient quality of diet (in micronutrients and/or macronutrients), the interplay between gut health, immune function and exposure to infectious disease [3], and occurs even in regions and households with apparent food security.

Wasted children are highly susceptible to disease and the risk of mortality increases substantially with the severity of the problem. The risk of dying among severely wasted children is 8–9 times higher than that of children with adequate weight [1]. Stunted children are also 4–5 times more likely to die from infectious diseases before their 5th birthday than children of adequate height. The total estimated number of stunted children (165 million in 2011) is almost an order of magnitude higher than the estimated number of severely wasted children (19 million in 2011) [4]. The actual number of child deaths due to stunting and associated complications is therefore higher than that due to wasting [1].

Stunting in the first 2–3 years of life results in lasting height deficits during adulthood with potential associated risks for women during childbearing years ultimately leading to intergenerational impacts on health and development [5]. Growth in the first 2 years of life is consistently associated with irreversible cognitive, motor and behavior development. In a number of settings, the effect size for poor cognitive scores among moderately to severely stunted children (height-for-age age z score <–2) compared to nonstunted children (z score >–1) was estimated to be moderate to high (0.4–1.05 standard deviation, SD) [6]. Malnutrition and neglect cause visible impairment to normal brain development (fig. 1) [7]. Interventions to improve nutrition and child growth during this early period translate into higher educational attainment [8] and improved human capital as adults [9].

In addition, there is ample evidence that healthy growth during the first 2 years of life will reduce the incidence of noncommunicable diseases in later life [10]. On the other hand, rapid weight gain without adequate length gain in early life may increase the risk of later obesity and cardiovascular disease risk factors [11]. The extent to which rapid infant growth represents a risk may depend on whether it occurs in the context of recovery from earlier growth restriction and results in normalization of bodyweight and length, or whether excess growth is predominantly ponderal with constrained linear gain, thus leading to excess weight-for-height [12]. Stunting can be an independent condition, or be present together with wasting. Stunting can even occur in the presence of overweight and obesity; the concept of stunted obesity reflects a true double burden of malnutrition [13, 14]. The risk of micronutrient deficiencies is elevated in all malnutrition conditions [12, 15, 16].

Neufeld · Osendarp

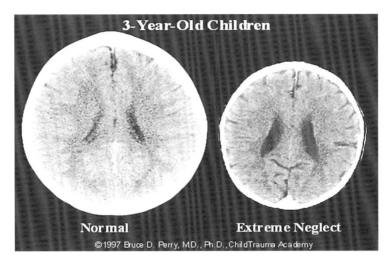

Fig. 1. Brain development in a child suffering from malnutrition compared to normal development. Reproduced with permission from Perry [7].

The Choice of Indicators to Track and Measure Progress on Nutrition

The inclusion of a nutrition indicator (weight-for-age) as a measure of progress for the Millennium Development Goals (MDGs) did much to position nutrition within the development agenda. Although vital for positioning, this indicator does little to provide clarity on the nature of the nutrition problems that must be addressed, the likely consequences, or specificity on the type of interventions that can be effective to address this. Wasting continues to be a vital indicator to target feeding programs and to assess progress towards its elimination in regions and countries. The World Health Assembly (WHA) has now endorsed a target of reducing and maintaining wasting at <5% globally by 2025 [17]. The importance of assessing linear growth is also well recognized, and the WHA targets include a 40% reduction in the prevalence of stunting by 2025.

With the increasing number of overweight adults and children even in developing countries, our measures of healthy growth should encompass not only height and insufficient weight, but also risk of excess weight; the WHA targets for 2025 call for no increase in childhood overweight by 2025. Healthy linear growth can be defined in comparison to 2006 WHO growth reference [3] and assessed using height and age at a population level. Healthy growth in weight, however, would require accurate assessment of changes in lean and fat body mass. While BMI is appropriate to identify adults at risk of disease, it may not be as useful in children because of their changing body shape [18, 19]. Furthermore, maturation pattern differs between genders and different ethnic groups [20], which adds to the problem of using BMI in children.

In research or clinical settings, a number of direct and proxy measures of body composition exist including underwater weighing (densitometry), multi-frequency bioelectrical impedance analysis, magnetic resonance imaging, and skinfold thickness. All of these require extensive training and/or costly equipment and are not appropriate for large-scale surveys in resource-poor environments. Waist circumference is now used extensively as a surrogate marker of visceral obesity in adults but is less well validated for children. A recent study of children 8–18 years of age has shown that after adjusting for age and sex, waist circumference-to-height ratio was a better predictor of variance in percent body fat (80%) than waist circumference alone (72%) or BMI (68%), with the sum of 2 skinfold thicknesses providing only a slightly better estimate (84%) [21]. Further research is needed to refine the measures of excess weight in children feasible for use in large population-based surveys.

Tracking Global and Regional Progress on Nutrition

Since the acceptance of the MDGs, the prevalence of undernutrition (low weight-for-age) has been tracked globally. According to the 2010 MDG report, the prevalence of underweight decreased at global level from 31 to 26% from 1990 to 2008; a rate of reduction which is not on track to reach the MDG of halving the number of underweight children by 2015 [22]. Inequities between urban and rural areas in most regions and variation in the extent of progress across regions are clearly identifiable using this indicator. For example, the ratio of underweight in rural compared to urban areas ranges from 1.2 in South East Asia for 4.8 in Eastern Asia. In Asia and Latin America, the ratio has increased (i.e. increased disparity between urban and rural areas), while in Africa there has been little change since 1990.

Recognizing the complexity of collecting and analyzing quality data, UNICEF, WHO and the World Bank have come together to harmonize data and statistical methods used to derive prevalence estimates of malnutrition in children and have updated prevalence estimates from 1990 to 2011 [4]. This includes reanalyzing (when possible) or adjusting prevalence estimates using the WHO 2006 reference standard and a standardized methodology for adjusting for variation in age across surveys and a single model to assess trends over time and region. Trends in child nutrition were also recently published by the Nutrition Impact Model Study Group [23]. This methodology permits taking into consideration the full range of nutritional deficiencies from mild to severe and allows for non-

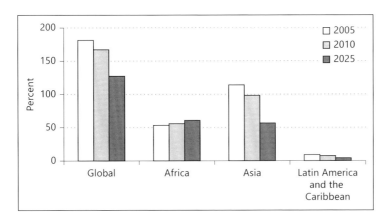

Fig. 2. Percentage of stunted children <5 years of age globally and by region in 2005, 2010 and estimated number in 2025 [24].

linear trends over time. Although the 2 methods result in slightly different prevalence estimates, the general conclusions with regard to trends across regions and over time are similar.

An updated summary of nutritional status of children globally using data from both reviews has recently been published as part of the updated Lancet Nutrition Series [24]. The data show that globally, the estimated number of stunted children is decreasing (fig. 2), but is not on track to meet the goal of 100 million by 2025. While substantial progress has been achieved in Asia, the prevalence of stunting is still high (over 25% in 2010), with almost 60% of all stunted children living in Asia. If current trends continue however, by 2025 the absolute number of stunted children in Africa will exceed that of Asia due to the very slow decline in prevalence in that region. From 1990 to 2010, the number of stunted children in Asia almost halved from 188.7 to 98.4 million, while in sub-Saharan Africa there was essentially no change in prevalence and the number of stunted children actually increased over the same period from 45.7 to 55.8 million.

There has been very little change in the absolute number of children suffering from severe wasting (weight-for-height z score <–3) since 2004, estimated at 3% or 19 million children globally. A total of 52 million children (8%) are estimated to suffer from moderate or severe wasting (weight-for-height z score <–2). On the contrary, there has been substantial increase in the number of overweight children, from 35.3 to 41.2 million, globally. The prevalence and number of overweight children has increased in Asia and Africa, and only in Latin America and the Caribbean has there been no substantial increase over the past years. The prevalence of overweight and obesity among children in the LAC region however is high and has increased substantially over the past decades.

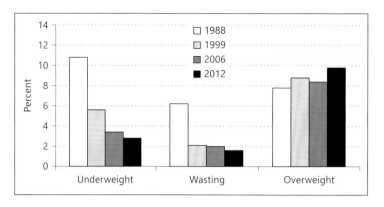

Fig. 3. Prevalence of underweight, wasting and overweight in children <5 years of age from 4 nationally representative surveys in Mexico [25]. Z scores estimated using 2006 WHO growth reference standard. Underweight: weight-for-age <2 SD below median; wasting: weight-for-height <2 SD below median; overweight: weight-for-height >2 SD above the median.

Nutritional Indicators as Measures of Inequity and Implications for Program Design

Although Latin America contributes only small numbers to the global burden, stunting is highly prevalent in some parts of the region and provides a powerful indicator of inequity within countries and across the region. For example, in Mexico, by 2006, wasting and underweight have ceased to be public health problems (<5%) even among the rural and indigenous populations [25] (fig. 3). Using these indicators, one might claim victory in combating undernutrition in this country. That conclusion however, would be very different using stunting. At a national level, the prevalence has declined substantially from 26.9% in 1988 to 13.6% in 2012. National level data however, hide enormous variation within the country reflective of substantial inequity. In figure 4, the prevalence of stunting among the most and least disadvantaged populations is contrasted. Among the most vulnerable populations living in poverty, in rural areas, particularly the rural south and among indigenous populations, the prevalence ranges from 20 to 34%. On the contrary, among those least disadvantaged, the prevalence ranges from 7 to 10%. This variation is not apparent in Mexico for indicators of weight; no substantial difference in the prevalence of wasting or overweight is evident among the different economic levels, urban versus rural populations with only small differences in the prevalence of overweight by region of the country (highest in the north).

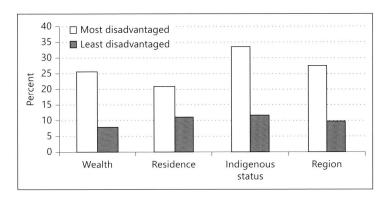

Fig. 4. Prevalence of stunting as evidence of inequity among the diverse population groups in Mexico, 2012 [25]. Most and least disadvantaged, respectively, defined as: wealth (lowest and highest quintile), residence (rural, urban), indigenous status (indigenous, nonindigenous) and region (rural southern region, rural northern region).

The data in Mexico provide clear priorities for the targeting of programs to address nutritional problems. Public health interventions are no longer needed in Mexico to address wasting. Efforts to improve linear growth and prevent stunting can be successfully targeted to those most at risk using economic criteria (lowest quintile) or region of residence, particularly the rural southern region. Social protection programs such as Mexico's Oportunidades that are effectively targeted to the poor [26] are therefore extremely well positioned as platforms for inclusion of nutrition actions. On the contrary, efforts to address excess weight are needed across all income groups and regions.

In countries with a higher burden of malnutrition, targeted approaches to reach those most at risk may be more costly than population-based programs. For example, a recent national survey in Pakistan reported a national prevalence of 43% stunting and 16.8% wasting [27]. Although differences exist within diverse groups in the country, the magnitude of those differences is much less striking than that observed in Mexico. For example, in urban areas of Pakistan, 36% of children are stunted and 13.9% wasted, while in rural areas, 45.9% are stunted and 18% wasted. Among the 7 provinces in the country, the prevalence of stunting ranges from 60 to 80%. For the purposes of decision making, such surveys should go beyond prevalence of specific health and nutrition outcomes and should assess the trends in determinants of poor nutrition such as breast and complementary feeding patterns, hygiene and sanitation that might increase the risk of infectious disease as well as program participation.

Conclusions

Recent global development movements are recognizing a clear need for indicators that can provide robust measures of trends in nutritional status of children, particularly during the critical first years of life. Such measures are needed by societies investing in nutrition to track progress and improve accountability and should be aspirational to mobilize sufficient investment in nutrition. At the same time, indicators of nutrition should be easy to understand and based on measurements that are feasible in population surveys. This can be done only by tracking problems of undernutrition, specifically stunting and wasting, and overweight. Recent global development goals call for tracking of all three indicators, but further investments in regular data collection will be required in many countries in order to achieve this.

Disclosure Statement

The authors declare that no financial or other conflict of interest exists in relation to the content of the chapter.

References

1   Black RE, Allen LH, Bhutta ZA, et al: Maternal and child undernutrition: global and regional exposures and health consequences. Lancet 2008;371:243–260.
2   Bhutta ZA, Ahmed T, Black RE, et al: What works? Interventions for maternal and child undernutrition and survival. Lancet 2008; 371:417–440.
3   Piwoz E, Sundberg S, Rooke J: Promoting healthy growth: what are the priorities for research and action? Adv Nutr 2012;3:234–241.
4   United Nations Children's Fund, World Health Organization, The World Bank: UNICEF-WHO-World Bank Joint Child Malnutrition Estimates. UNICEF, New York, WHO, Geneva, The World Bank, Washington, 2012.
5   Martorell R, Zongrone A: Intergenerational influences on child growth and undernutrition. Paediatr Perinat Epidemiol 2012; 26(suppl 1):302–314.
6   Grantham-McGregor S, Cheung YB, Cueto S, et al: Developmental potential in the first 5 years for children in developing countries. Lancet 2007;369:60–70.
7   Perry BD: Childhood experience and the expression of genetic potential: what childhood neglect tells us about nature and nurture. Brain Mind 2002;3:79–100.
8   Martorell R, Horta BL, Adair LS, et al: Weight gain in the first two years of life is an important predictor of schooling outcomes in pooled analyses from five birth cohorts from low- and middle-income countries. J Nutr 2010;140:348–354.
9   Martorell R, Melgar P, Maluccio JA, et al: The nutrition intervention improved adult human capital and economic productivity. J Nutr 2010;140:411–414.
10 Victora CG, Adair L, Fall C, et al: Maternal and child undernutrition: consequences for adult health and human capital. Lancet 2008; 371:340–357.

11 Monteiro PO, Victora CG: Rapid growth in infancy and childhood and obesity in later life – a systematic review. Obes Rev 2005;6: 143–154.

12 Uauy R, Corvalan C, Dangour AD: Conference on 'Multidisciplinary approaches to nutritional problems'. Rank Prize Lecture. Global nutrition challenges for optimal health and well-being. Proc Nutr Soc 2009; 68:34–42.

13 Uauy R, Kain J, Mericq V, et al: Nutrition, child growth, and chronic disease prevention. Ann Med 2008;40:11–20.

14 Shetty P: Community-based approaches to address childhood undernutrition and obesity in developing countries; in Kalhan SC, Prentice AM, Yajnik CS (eds): Emerging Societies – Coexistence of Childhood Malnutrition and Obesity. Nestlé Nutr Workshop Ser Pediatr Program. Vevey, Nestec/Basel, Karger, 2009, vol 63, pp 227–254.

15 Aeberli I, Hurrell RF, Zimmermann MB: Overweight children have higher circulating hepcidin concentrations and lower iron status but have dietary iron intakes and bioavailability comparable with normal weight children. Int J Obes (Lond) 2009;33:1111–1117.

16 Aeberli I, Biebinger R, Lehmann R, et al: Serum retinol-binding protein 4 concentration and its ratio to serum retinol are associated with obesity and metabolic syndrome components in children. J Clin Endocrinol Metab 2007;92:4359–4365.

17 World Health Organization: Sixty-fifth World Health Assembly. Resolutions and Decisions. Annex 2 (2012). http://apps.who.int/gb/ebwha/pdf_files/WHA65-REC1/A65_REC1-en.pdf.

18 World Health Organization: Methods and Development, WHO Child Growth Standards: Length/Height-for-Age, Weight-for-Age, Weight-for-Length, Weight-for-Height and Body Mass Index-for-Age. Geneva, World Health Organization, 2006.

19 Cole TJ, Bellizzi MC, Flegal KM, et al: Establishing a standard definition for child overweight and obesity worldwide: international survey. BMJ 2000;320:1240–1243.

20 Wang Y: Epidemiology of childhood obesity – methodological aspects and guidelines: what is new? Int J Obesity 2004;28:S21–S28.

21 Brambilla P, Bedogni G, Heo M, et al: Waist circumference-to-height ratio predicts adiposity better than body mass index in children and adolescents. Int J Obes (Lond) DOI: 10.1038/ijo.2013.32.

22 United Nations Department of Economic and Social Affairs (DESA): The Millennium Development Goals Report, June 2010. www.un.org/millenniumgoals.

23 Stevens GA, Finucane MM, Paciorek CJ, et al: Trends in mild, moderate, and severe stunting and underweight, and progress towards MDG 1 in 141 developing countries: a systematic analysis of population representative data. Lancet 2012;380:824–834.

24 Black RE, Victora CG, Walker SP, et al: Maternal and child undernutrition and overweight in low-income and middle-income countries. Lancet 2013;382:427–451.

25 Rivera Dommarco JA, Cuevas Nasu L, González de Cossío T, et al: Chronic malnutrition in Mexico in the last quarter century: recommendations for its virtual elimination (in Spanish). Salud Pub Mex, in press.

26 Gaarder MM, Glassman A, Todd JE: Conditional cash transfers and health: unpacking the causal chain. J Develop Effectiveness 2010;2:6–50.

27 Aga Khan University: National Nutrition Survey. Karachi, Aga Khan University, 2011.

Black RE, Singhal A, Uauy R (eds): International Nutrition: Achieving Millennium Goals and Beyond.
Nestlé Nutr Inst Workshop Ser, vol 78, pp 21–28, (DOI: 10.1159/000354932)
Nestec Ltd., Vevey/S. Karger AG., Basel, © 2014

Global Distribution and Disease Burden Related to Micronutrient Deficiencies

Robert E. Black

Bloomberg School of Public Health, Johns Hopkins University, Baltimore, MD, USA

Abstract

Micronutrients are vitamins and minerals that are essential for human life and health. Deficiencies in these micronutrients are common because of poor quality diets and frequent infectious diseases in low- and middle-income countries. The high prevalence of deficiencies and their important adverse consequences on mortality, morbidity and disability result in a substantial disease burden. In particular, deficiencies of vitamin A and zinc increase the risk of child mortality, and zinc deficiency increases infectious morbidity and reduces linear growth as well. Deficiencies of iodine and iron are significant primarily for their effects on development and cognition and consequent disabilities. Programs targeting each of these micronutrients are underway and, particularly for vitamin A and iodine, have some success. Greater efforts to address these and the full set of micronutrients are needed to reduce their global burden of diseases.

© 2014 Nestec Ltd., Vevey/S. Karger AG, Basel

Introduction

Essential vitamins and minerals, referred to collectively as micronutrients, have critical roles in human metabolism, immunity and other body functions. The deficiency of some can cause a unique clinical syndrome, yet it is the more insidious effects of some of the micronutrients that have the greatest effects on health and human capacity. Even as the classical clinical manifestations have diminished, the deficiencies of many vitamins and minerals have persisted with important adverse consequences, especially in low- and middle-income countries. This review will focus on the deficiencies of selected micronutrients because of their important global distribution and disease burden, namely vitamin A, zinc, iodine and iron.

Vitamin A Deficiency

The characteristic clinical feature of vitamin A deficiency is xerophthalmia, with severity ranging from night blindness to corneal ulceration keratomalacia, leading to corneal scarring and possibly blindness. The more severe forms of xerophthalmia are now very infrequent, possibly due to additional vitamin A intake, especially from programs that provide high-dose supplements every 6 months as well as control of measles and other infectious diseases that may precipitate the clinical conditions. However, night blindness continues to be common in some populations. The World Health Organization (WHO) estimates that 7.8% (7.0–8.7%) of pregnant women are afflicted with night blindness, affecting nearly 10 million women worldwide [1]. Vitamin A deficiency is also assessed by serum retinol concentrations with <0.70 μmol/l indicating deficiency. WHO estimates that 15.3% (7.4–23.2%) of pregnant women have subclinical deficiency, affecting 19 million women. Pre-school children are also at risk of vitamin A deficiency. WHO estimates the global prevalence of night blindness to be 0.9% (0.3–1.5%), affecting 5 million children, and the prevalence of subclinical deficiency based on serum retinol concentrations to be 33.3% (31.1–35.4%), affecting 90 million children [1].

Maternal night blindness has been associated with increased rates of babies born with low birthweight and with infant mortality [2, 3]. The relationship of maternal vitamin A deficiency with these outcomes, as studied in supplementation trials in pregnancy, has not been found to be significant when the three trials are combined; however, subclinical vitamin A deficiency in children has important consequences for mortality. A meta-analysis of the trials of vitamin A supplementation found a 23% reduction in deaths in the 6–59 months age group, a statistically significant benefit for diarrhea deaths and a suggestive one for measles deaths [4].

We calculated the deaths that could be attributed to vitamin A deficiency using estimated deaths due to diarrhea and measles in 2011 [5]. The risk of vitamin A deficiency was said to be the inverse of the trial effects on these two causes of death, adjusted with the assumption that all of the effect was in the subset of the population that had subclinical deficiency in the trial populations. This adjusted relative risk was then applied to the current prevalence of subclinical deficiency. The estimated deaths for 2011 attributed to current vitamin A deficiency is

157,000, two thirds of which would be in Africa and nearly all of the rest in Asia. Nearly all of these deaths were related to diarrhea, because measles deaths are low due to extensive vaccination programs.

Zinc Deficiency

Zinc is an essential mineral with many biological functions in humans. The characteristic clinical features of rash, alopecia, hypogonadism and reduced immunocompetence occur with severe dietary zinc deficiency and with acrodermatitis enteropathica, a genetic defect in zinc absorption, but these are rarely seen. Instead, subclinical zinc deficiency that does not have overt manifestations of deficiency but does have important consequences is common. Recent estimates based on analysis of national food balances suggest that 17% of the world's population may consume a diet that has inadequate amounts of bioavailable zinc [6]. Based on dietary intakes in pregnancy, it has also been estimated that as many as 82% of pregnant women may have inadequate zinc intakes [7]. Likewise, pre-school children may have prevalences of zinc deficiency higher than the population average because of their limited consumption of animal-source foods and the cereal-based complementary food diets containing phytates that reduce the bioavailability of zinc.

Severe zinc deficiency in pregnancy is associated with fetal growth restriction, preterm delivery and maternal morbidity, including hemorrhage [8, 9]. A recent systematic review of randomized controlled trials found that women who received zinc supplements in pregnancy had a 14% reduction in preterm deliveries [10]. Subclinical zinc deficiency in children is associated with increased incidence rates of and mortality from diarrhea, pneumonia and possibly other infectious diseases. Because observational studies are unable to discern causal relationships with the common childhood diseases, a number of randomized controlled trials have been done and subjected to meta-analyses. A recent review found that zinc-supplemented pre-school children had a 9% reduction in all-cause mortality (RR 0.91, 95% CI 0.82–1.01) of borderline statistical significance [11]. Another analysis of available trials found an 18% reduction in deaths in children 12–59 months of age (RR 0.82, 95% CI 0.70–0.96) [12]. In these meta-analyses, there were suggestive benefits for diarrhea mortality (RR 0.82, 95% CI 0.64–1.05) and pneumonia mortality (RR 0.85, 95% CI 0.65–1.11) [11]. There were also statistically significant reductions in diarrhea incidence (RR 0.87, 95% CI 0.81–0.94) and pneumonia incidence (RR 0.81, 95% CI 0.73–0.90). Zinc deficiency also reduces linear growth in young children [11].

To estimate the deaths attributed to zinc deficiency in children, we used the inverse of the reductions in cause-specific mortality in children 1–4 years old adjusted with the assumption that all the benefit was in the subset of the trial populations that was at risk of zinc deficiency based on the availability of zinc in national diets [5, 6]. This adjusted risk estimate was then applied to the current estimated prevalence of inadequate zinc intake in countries. It is estimated that for 2011 116,065 child deaths, about equally split between diarrhea and pneumonia, could be attributed to zinc deficiency; 57% of the deaths were in Africa and 42% in Asia.

Iodine Deficiency

Severe iodine deficiency during pregnancy causes cretinism [13]. In addition, studies done in highly endemic areas of iodine deficiency found average deficits of about 13 IQ points in the offspring of mothers likely to have been iodine deficient in pregnancy [14, 15]. It is questionable if less severe levels of iodine deficiency have an effect on brain development and cognition [16, 17].

The measure of iodine deficiency is a population one not an individual one. The median urinary iodine concentration in school-age children is used to assess the iodine status of a population. Median values of <100 μg/l are considered to represent deficiency. Iodine requirements increase 50% in pregnancy, and deficiency is defined as <150 μg/l for a population of pregnant women; however, the data from children are largely used to establish national and global prevalences of deficiency. Recent estimates are that 28.7% of the world's population, in some regions up to 50%, or 1.9 billion people are deficient [16–18]. This is largely mild deficiency, the consequences of which are unclear, but there may be some individuals still who have severe deficiency in spite of widespread use of iodized salt to increase intake.

Iodine deficiency rarely causes death, but it can result in disability. Our previous estimates were that in 2004 it resulted in a loss of 2.6 million disability-adjusted life years (DALYs) or 0.5% of the DALYS in children under 5 years old [19]. New estimates from the Global Burden of Disease Project are that iodine deficiency resulted in a loss of 4.0 million DALYs in 2010 [20].

Iron Deficiency

Iron deficiency as a cause of anemia is globally prevalent. We estimate that the prevalence of anemia that responds to iron supplementation (referred to hereafter as iron deficiency anemia or IDA) ranges from 11 to 16% for pre-school children and 10–15% for pregnant women for UN regions, the highest prevalence in Africa followed closely by Asia (table 1) [5].

Table 1. Prevalence (%) of deficiencies of selected micronutrients by UN regions

UN region	Vitamin A deficiency				Zinc deficiency	Iodine deficiency	Iron deficiency anemia	
	children <5 years		pregnant women		children 6–12 years	total population	children <5 years	pregnant women
	night blind	serum retinol <0.70 µmol/l	night blind	serum retinol <0.70 µmol/l	urine iodine <100 µg/l	National diet inadequate in zinc	hemoglobin <110 g/l	hemoglobin <110 g/l
Africa	2.1	41.6	9.4	14.3	39.4	23.9	16.4	17.2
Americas	0.6	15.6	4.4	2.0	13.7	9.6	11.5	13.7
Asia	0.5	33.5	7.8	18.4	28.4	19.4	15.7	16.3
Europe	0.7	14.9	2.9	2.2	45.5	7.6	10.8	14.6
Oceania	0.5	12.6	9.2	1.4	53.7	5.7	13.2	15.4

Maternal anemia is a risk factor for death during labor and delivery. A recent analysis of 10 observational studies found an odds ratio of 0.71 (95% CI 0.60–0.85) for maternal mortality for a 10 g/l increase in hemoglobin in pregnancy [21]. There is a possible link between maternal IDA and adverse birth outcomes. A meta-analysis of 11 trials of iron or iron/folic acid supplementation in pregnancy found a statistically significant 20% (RR 0.80, 95% CI 0.71–0.90) lower rate of low birthweight in the iron versus control group; rates of small for gestational age or preterm births were not significantly different [22]. Trials also find a reduction in neonatal and child mortality in offspring of iron-supplemented mothers during pregnancy [23, 24]. On the other hand, iron supplementation in childhood appears to have no mortality benefit.

Maternal iron supplementation may have other benefits for maternal mental health and maternal-child relations, perhaps related to reduced fatigue [25, 26]. Maternal iron supplementation may also benefit the offspring's development, including IQ and executive functioning at school age [27, 28].

Iron supplementation in school-aged children with IDA generally benefits their cognition, but in pre-school children this has not been demonstrated [29–31]. Of 7 randomized, controlled trials of iron supplementation in young children, only one found a benefit in mental development, while 5 showed benefits in motor development [32–39].

There are very few deaths in children that could be attributed to iron deficiency or IDA, so the estimation of disease burden depends on the disability from anemia. Our previous estimate for the disease burden in children was a loss of about 2 million DALYs in 2004 [19]. The recent Global Burden of Disease Project estimate is about 15 million childhood DALYs [20].

Implications for Nutrition Programs

Deficiencies of vitamin A, zinc, iodine and iron, among all the possible deficiencies of micronutrients deserve focus because they have a high global prevalence and important health effects. These deficiencies may coexist in populations and even in individuals with deficiencies of other vitamins and minerals. Of note in this regard is that poor folate status at the time of conception may lead to neural tube defects in the fetus, particularly in women who are genetically susceptible and thus need more folate. Deficiencies of some of the B vitamins and vitamin D may also have adverse effects on women in pregnancy, on the fetus and on the young child and are subjects of active investigation.

There are programs in low- and middle-income countries to reduce these micronutrient deficiencies or ameliorate their negative effects. Supplementation with high-dose vitamin A reaches a high proportion of children living in areas with deficient diets. As a result, the number of deaths attributed to vitamin A deficiency is reduced; however, without continued intervention, the deaths would increase because the dietary inadequacy has not been corrected except in a few countries with food fortification programs. Zinc is now recommended for use in treatment of childhood diarrhea, and as coverage increases, this should have benefits both for treatment of that episode of illness and for prevention of subsequent infectious diseases. It would still be desirable to have programs that increase the consumption of zinc in the diet or provide zinc supplements to vulnerable age groups including pregnant women and young children. Iodine deficiency is being addressed primarily through programs to fortify salt with iodine, and this is now reaching more than 70% of the world's population [40]. IDA remains a problem with only limited programmatic efforts. Iron and folic acid is to be taken by all pregnant women, but the adherence to this recommendation is low. Iron supplementation in children is increasing through the use of micronutrient powders and fortified products, but coverage is still very low.

Given the possible occurrence of a number of micronutrient deficiencies, the limited data on the distribution of deficiencies in populations and the difficulty of diagnosing deficiencies in individuals, additional efforts are needed. There is increasing evidence on the value of giving a multiple micronutrient supplement in pregnancy instead of iron and folic acid. Similarly, there would be value in approaches that ensure dietary adequacy of micronutrients, as well as calories, protein and essential fatty acids, possibly through fortification of foods for specific target population groups such as young children.

The disease burden caused by micronutrient deficiencies is substantial, but completely preventable. More precise quantification of the prevalence of these deficiencies within countries and in vulnerable groups should guide the interventions available and encourage innovative approaches. Better assessment of the consequences, throughout the life course, of these deficiencies may help to motivate action and give greater priority to nutritional interventions and programs.

Disclosure Statement

R.E. Black is a member of the governing boards of the Micronutrient Initiative and Vitamin Angels.

References

1 World Health Organization: Global prevalence of vitamin A deficiency in populations at risk 1995–2005: WHO global database on vitamin A deficiency. World Health Organization, Geneva, 2009, pp 10–11.
2 Christian P, West KP Jr, Khatry SK, et al: Maternal night blindness increases risk of mortality in the first 6 months of life among infants in Nepal. J Nutr 2001;131:1510–1512.
3 Tielsch JM, Rahmathullah L, Katz J, et al: Maternal night blindness during pregnancy is associated with low birthweight, morbidity, and poor growth in South India. J Nutr 2008; 138:787–792.
4 Beaton GH, Martorell R, Aronson KJ, et al, Administrative Committee on Coordination/ Subcommittee on Nutrition: Effectiveness of vitamin A supplementation in the control of young child morbidity and mortality in developing countries. Nutrition Policy Discussion Paper 13. Geneva, United Nations, 1993.
5 Black RE, Victora CG, Walker SP, et al, the Maternal and Child Nutrition Study Group: Maternal and child undernutrition and overweight in low- and middle-income countries. Lancet 2013;382:427–451.
6 Wessells KR, Brown KH: Estimating the global prevalence of zinc deficiency: results based on zinc availability in national food supplies and the prevalence of stunting. PloS One 2012;7:e50568.
7 Shils ME, Shike M: Modern Nutrition in Health and Disease. Philadelphia, Lippincott Williams & Wilkins, 2005.
8 King JC: Determinants of maternal zinc status during pregnancy. Am J Clin Nutr 2000; 71:1334s–1343s.
9 Simmer K, Thompson RP: Maternal zinc and intrauterine growth retardation. Clin Sci (Lond) 1985;68:395–399.
10 Mori R, Ota E, Middleton P, et al: Zinc supplementation for improving pregnancy and infant outcome. Cochrane Database Syst Rev 2012;7:CD000230.
11 Yakoob MY, Theodoratou E, Jabeen A, et al: Preventive zinc supplementation in developing countries: impact on mortality and morbidity due to diarrhea, pneumonia and malaria. BMC Public Health 2011;11(suppl 3):S23.
12 Brown KH, Peerson JM, Baker SK, Hess SY: Preventive zinc supplementation among infants, preschoolers, and older prepubertal children. Food Nutr Bull 2009;30(suppl 1):12S–40S.
13 Pharoah P, Buttfield I, Hetzel B: Neurological damage to the fetus resulting from severe iodine deficiency during pregnancy. Lancet 1971;297:308–310.
14 Bleichrodt N, Born MP: A Meta-Analysis of Research on Iodine and Its Relationship to Cognitive Development. The Damaged Brain of Iodine Deficiency. New York, Cognizant Communication, 1994, pp 195–200.
15 Qian M, Wang D, Watkins WE, et al: The effects of iodine on intelligence in children: a meta-analysis of studies conducted in China. Asia Pac J Clin Nutr 2005;14:32–42.
16 Skeaff SA: Iodine deficiency in pregnancy: the effect on neurodevelopment in the child. Nutrients 2011;3:265–273.
17 Zimmermann MB, Andersson M: Assessment of iodine nutrition in populations: past, present, and future. Nutr Rev 2012;70:553–570.
18 Andersson M, Karumbunathan V, Zimmermann MB: Global iodine status in 2011 and trends over the past decade. J Nutr 2012;142:744–750.

19 Black RE, Allen LH, Bhutta ZA, et al, Maternal and Child Undernutrition Study Group: Maternal and child undernutrition: global and regional exposures and health consequences. Lancet 2008;371:243–260.

20 Lim SS, Vos T, Flaxman AD, et al: A comparative risk assessment of burden of disease and injury attributable to 67 risk factors and risk factor clusters in 21 regions, 1990–2010: a systematic analysis for the Global Burden of Disease Study 2010. Lancet 2013;380:2224–2260.

21 Murray-Kolb LE, Chen L, Chen P, et al: CHERG Iron Report: Maternal Mortality, Child Mortality, Perinatal Mortality, Child Cognition, and Estimates of Prevalence of Anemia due to Iron Deficiency. Baltimore, CHERG, 2012.

22 Imdad A, Bhutta ZA: Routine iron/folate supplementation during pregnancy: effect on maternal anaemia and birth outcomes. Paediatr Perinat Epidemiol 2012;26(suppl 1):168–177.

23 Christian P, Stewart CP, LeClerq SC, et al: Antenatal and postnatal iron supplementation and childhood mortality in rural Nepal: a prospective follow-up in a randomized, controlled community trial. Am J Epidemiol 2009;170:1127–1136.

24 Zeng L, Dibley MJ, Cheng Y, et al: Impact of micronutrient supplementation during pregnancy on birth weight, duration of gestation, and perinatal mortality in rural western China: double blind cluster randomised controlled trial. BMJ 2008;337:a2001.

25 Beard JL, Hendricks MK, Perez EM, et al: Maternal iron deficiency anemia affects postpartum emotions and cognition. J Nutr 2005; 135:267–272.

26 Murray-Kolb LE: Iron status and neuropsychological consequences in women of reproductive age: what do we know and where are we headed? J Nutr 2011;141:747S–755S.

27 Christian P, Murray-Kolb LE, Khatry SK, et al: Prenatal micronutrient supplementation and intellectual and motor function in early school-aged children in Nepal. JAMA 2010; 304:2716–2723.

28 Perez EM, Hendricks MK, Beard JL, et al: Mother-infant interactions and infant development are altered by maternal iron deficiency anemia. J Nutr 2005;135:850–855.

29 Grantham-McGregor S, Baker-Henningham H: Iron deficiency in childhood: causes and consequences for child development. Ann Nestle 2010;68:105–119.

30 Sachdev H, Gera T, Nestel P: Effect of iron supplementation on mental and motor development in children: systematic review of randomised controlled trials. Public Health Nutr 2005;8:117–132.

31 Szajewska H, Ruszczynski M, Chmielewska A: Effects of iron supplementation in nonanemic pregnant women, infants, and young children on the mental performance and psychomotor development of children: a systematic review of randomized controlled trials. Am J Clin Nutr 2010;91:1684–1690.

32 Maternal anthropometry and pregnancy outcomes. A WHO Collaborative Study. Bull World Health Organ 1995;73:1S–98S.

33 Aukett M, Parks YA, Scott PH, Wharton BA: Treatment with iron increases weight gain and psychomotor development. Arch Dis Child 1986;61:849–857.

34 Black MM, Baqui AH, Zaman K, et al: Iron and zinc supplementation promote motor development and exploratory behavior among Bangladeshi infants. Am J Clin Nutr 2004;80:903–910.

35 Friel JK, Aziz K, Andrews WL, et al: A double-masked, randomized control trial of iron supplementation in early infancy in healthy term breast-fed infants. J Pediatr 2003;143:582–586.

36 Idjradinata P, Pollitt E: Reversal of developmental delays in iron-deficient anaemic infants treated with iron. Lancet 1993;341:1–4.

37 Lind T, Lönnerdal B, Stenlund H, et al: A community-based randomized controlled trial of iron and zinc supplementation in Indonesian infants: interactions between iron and zinc. Am J Clin Nutr 2003;77:883–890.

38 Moffatt M, Longstaffe S, Besant J, Dureski C: Prevention of iron deficiency and psychomotor decline in high-risk infants through use of iron-fortified infant formula: a randomized clinical trial. J Pediatr 1994;125:527–534.

39 Stoltzfus RJ, Kvalsvig JD, Chwaya HM, et al: Effects of iron supplementation and anthelmintic treatment on motor and language development of preschool children in Zanzibar: double blind, placebo controlled study. BMJ 2001;323:1389–1393.

40 Campbell N, Dary O, Cappuccio FP, et al: Collaboration to optimize dietary intakes of salt and iodine: a critical but overlooked public health issue. Bull World Health Organ 2012;90:73–74.

Black RE, Singhal A, Uauy R (eds): International Nutrition: Achieving Millennium Goals and Beyond.
Nestlé Nutr Inst Workshop Ser, vol 78, pp 29–38, (DOI: 10.1159/000355056)
Nestec Ltd., Vevey/S. Karger AG., Basel, © 2014

Predicting the Health Effects of Switching Infant Feeding Practices for Use in Decision-Making

Benjamin O. Yarnoff[a] · Benjamin T. Allaire[a] · Patrick Detzel[b]

[a]Public Health Economics Program, RTI International, Research Triangle Park, NC, USA;
[b]Nestlé Research Center, Lausanne, Switzerland

Abstract

Research has been plentiful to show pediatricians and public health practitioners the importance of exclusive breastfeeding for infant health. However, this past research is lacking in a few ways that are important for pediatricians and public health practitioners: it rarely examines broad geographies, and so cannot be generalized for different countries, it does not quantify the predicted effects of infant feeding, and it does not examine the effects of a range of feeding practices on infant health, instead focusing solely on exclusive breastfeeding. The present research simulates the effect on infant health of switching between a range of feeding practices using data from many countries. The results provide quantified estimates of the effect of switching between specific feeding practices such as exclusive breastfeeding, breastfeeding supplemented with milk liquids, or breastfeeding supplemented with solid foods and nonmilk liquids, as well as others. These quantified estimates of the effect of switching infant feeding practices can be used by pediatricians to motivate individual decisions about infant feeding and by public health practitioners and policymakers to motivate infant feeding programs and policy. Through these channels, they can hopefully play a role in improving infant health.

© 2014 Nestec Ltd., Vevey/S. Karger AG, Basel

Introduction

Research has been plentiful to show pediatricians and public health practitioners the importance of exclusive breastfeeding for infant health [1–9]. Furthermore, the World Health Organization and UNICEF recommend exclusive breastfeeding to 6 months of age, with continued breastfeeding along with appropriate complementary foods to 2 years of age or beyond [10]. However, this past research is lacking in a few ways that are important for pediatricians and public health practitioners. First, they do not examine broad geographies and so they cannot be generalized for decisions about infants in different countries. Because of this, they rarely quantify the predicted effects of infant feeding in a manner that can be used for addressing infant feeding practices across the world. Finally, past research has rarely examined the effects of a range of feeding practices on infant health, instead focusing solely on exclusive breastfeeding. This is perhaps the most important omission practically for pediatricians and public health practitioners, because a majority of infants in developing countries receive a wide range of foods in addition to breast milk [11, 12]. If different foods have different effects on infant health, then it is important for decision-makers to have a quantified rank ordering of potential feeding practices.

Yarnoff et al. [12] previously examined the association between a range of foods and infant health using regression analysis. In that research, the authors used simulation analysis to quantify the effect of switching between a few basic feeding practices such as nonexclusive breastfeeding supplemented with solid foods and exclusive breastfeeding. In the present research, we used the estimated associations from that regression analysis to simulate the effect of switching between a wider range of feeding practices. This expanded simulation provides practitioners with quantified estimates of the effects of switching between a variety of feeding practices that they can use in their work to improve infant health.

Methods

We simulate the health effects of switching between a range of infant feeding practices using estimated associations between six food categories and infant health from past research we conducted [12]. In this past research, we took data from the Demographic Health Survey (DHS) in 20 countries for multiple years (54 total surveys). The DHS is a nationally representative survey of women aged 15–49 that is funded by USAID, receives technical support from the US Census Bureau, and is conducted in developing countries approximately every 5 years. The survey asks about the health of each woman and her children as well as demographics and socioeconomics and all foods that the woman's youngest child was given in the past 24 h. The sample used in this analysis and our past analysis consists of 37,750 infants aged 0–6 months.

We decided ex-ante to examine 20 countries from the Africa, Asia, Latin America regions and selected these countries based on the following criteria: multiple survey years per country and the presence of information on infant feeding and maternal characteristics in each survey. Countries were selected to maximize these two criteria while also maintaining a distribution across the regions. The full DHS sample contains approximately 145,000 infants aged 0–6 months compared with 37,750 in our subsample. We tested the subsample for the representativeness of the full sample of DHS surveys by comparing mean measures of breastfeeding for infants aged 0–6 months, under-5 mortality, and diarrhea incidence between our subsample and the full sample (taken from the DHS website). Mean indicators were virtually identical between this subsample and the full sample of DHS surveys for exclusive breastfeeding among infants 0–6 months old (35% in the full sample and 33% in the subsample), nonexclusive breastfeeding among infants 0–6 months old (61% in the full sample and 63% in the subsample), under-5 mortality in the past 5 years (99 per 1,000 in the full sample and 101 per 1,000 in the subsample), and diarrhea incidence (20% in the full sample and 21% in the subsample). These similarities suggest that this subsample is representative of overall feeding practices in the full DHS sample and that results are generalizable across the full geography of the DHS.

We conducted regression analysis with community fixed effects and individual and family control variables estimating the association between six food types (exclusive breastfeeding, nonexclusive breastfeeding, solid foods, infant formula, milk liquids, and nonmilk liquids) and seven infant health measures (length-for-age z score, weight-for-height z score, stunted, wasted, diarrhea in the past 2 weeks, cough in the past 2 weeks, and fever in the past 2 weeks). In our initial research, we used these estimated associations to simulate the effects of switching to exclusive breastfeeding of a small set of feeding practices, nonexclusive breastfeeding with only one other food (infant formula, solid food, milk liquids, or nonmilk liquids). In the present research, we examined a larger set of feeding practices and also examined the effect of switching to feeding practices other than exclusive breastfeeding. This expanded simulation analysis provides important information to practitioners on the large set of feeding practices that they see in infants and helps quantify the rank order of alternative feeding practices for women who will never choose exclusive breastfeeding for their infants.

To simulate the effect of switching between feeding practices, we use the regression coefficients from Yarnoff et al. [12] to predict health levels in the DHS subsample for 10 different behaviors: exclusive breastfeeding and nonexclusive breastfeeding supplemented with either solids only, liquid milk only, infant formula only, nonmilk liquids only, nonmilk liquids and solids, nonmilk liquids and formula, nonmilk liquids and milk liquids, milk liquids and formula, and milk liquids and solids. The effect of switching to an alternative feeding practice was estimated as the difference between two practices. All estimates were conducted using the sample-weighted averages of the covariates in the regression and were bootstrapped 1,000 times to provide 95% confidence intervals.

Results

Our simulation analysis shows that infant health improves when switching to exclusive breastfeeding regardless of the initial feeding practice (table 1). The positive effect on health is present for six of the seven measures of infant health. Only wasting is not improved by switching to exclusive breastfeeding. Of great interest in the simulated effects of switching to exclusive breastfeeding are the magnitudes of the effect for each initial feeding practice. Table 1 includes re-

Table 1. Simulated effects of switching to exclusive breastfeeding, age 0–6 months

Starting feeding practice	Length z score	Weight z score	Stunted
NEBF + solids	0.138 (0.022 to 0.255)*	0.174 (0.060 to 0.288)*	–0.039 (–0.070 to –0.009)*
NEBF + milk liquids	0.160 (0.055 to 0.266)*	0.115 (0.012 to 0.218)*	–0.023 (–0.050 to 0.004)
NEBF + nonmilk liquids	0.119 (0.056 to 0.182)*	0.058 (–0.018 to 0.135)	–0.015 (–0.030 to 0.000)*
NEBF + infant formula	0.249 (0.098 to 0.401)*	0.064 (–0.083 to 0.212)	–0.028 (–0.065 to 0.008)
NEBF + nonmilk liquids + milk liquids	0.127 (0.042 to 0.211)*	0.159 (0.077 to 0.241)*	–0.021 (–0.042 to 0.000)*
NEBF + nonmilk liquids + solids	0.104 (0.029 to 0.180)*	0.218 (0.134 to 0.303)*	–0.038 (–0.056 to –0.019)*
NEBF + milk liquids + solids	0.146 (0.034 to 0.258)*	0.275 (0.167 to 0.382)*	–0.045 (–0.074 to –0.016)*
NEBF + milk liquids + infant formula	0.257 (0.108 to 0.406)*	0.165 (0.020 to 0.310)*	–0.034 (–0.072 to –0.004)
NEBF + nonmilk liquids + infant formula	0.216 (0.088 to 0.343)*	0.109 (–0.019 to 0.236)	–0.027 (–0.056 to 0.003)

NEBF = Nonexclusive breastfeeding. Confidence intervals are presented in parentheses and based on 1,000 bootstrapped replications of regression analysis. * $p < 0.05$.

sults presented in Yarnoff et al. [12] in order to compare the magnitude of effects across feeding practices. An examination of the results shows that some practices see greater benefits from switching to exclusive breastfeeding than others.

Simulations also show that there are health benefits for switching from some feeding practices to breast milk supplemented with milk liquids (table 2). These effects are seen in reducing the prevalence of diarrhea, cough, and fever. It is only beneficial to switch to feeding breast milk and milk liquids if the initial feeding practice included solid foods. Switching from other feeding practices may have positive or negative estimated effects, but these estimates are not statistically significant. For example, in the case of breastfeeding supplemented with infant formula, switching to supplementation with milk liquids has some negative and some positive effects, but these are statistically insignificant due to large variation coming from a small sample of infants receiving infant formula. Again, it is of great interest to see the magnitude of these simulated effects, especially for those that are statistically significant.

Wasted	Diarrhea	Fever	Cough
−0.046 (−0.095 to 0.002)	−0.083 (−0.115 to −0.050)*	−0.124 (−0.164 to −0.084)*	−0.107 (−0.150 to −0.064)*
−0.048 (−0.095 to −0.001)*	−0.006 (−0.033 to 0.022)	−0.068 (−0.100 to −0.036)*	−0.059 (−0.097 to −0.022)*
−0.008 (−0.032 to 0.017)	−0.046 (−0.062 to −0.030)*	−0.062 (−0.080 to −0.043)*	−0.040 (−0.060 to −0.020)*
−0.009 (−0.026 to 0.007)	−0.028 (−0.069 to 0.013)	−0.052 (−0.101 to −0.003)*	−0.050 (−0.104 to 0.004)
−0.002 (−0.020 to 0.017)	−0.029 (−0.051 to −0.006)*	−0.082 (−0.109 to −0.055)*	−0.060 (−0.088 to −0.031)*
0.007 (−0.012 to 0.026)	−0.106 (−0.126 to −0.086)*	−0.138 (−0.161 to −0.114)*	−0.107 (−0.133 to −0.081)*
0.000 (−0.020 to 0.020)	−0.065 (−0.095 to −0.035)*	−0.144 (−0.181 to −0.108)*	−0.127 (−0.168 to −0.086)*
0.004 (−0.009 to 0.016)	−0.011 (−0.050 to 0.029)	−0.073 (−0.121 to −0.025)*	−0.070 (−0.123 to −0.016)*
0.012 (−0.011 to 0.034)	−0.051 (−0.087 to −0.015)*	−0.066 (−0.109 to −0.023)*	−0.050 (−0.097 to −0.004)*

The simulation analysis demonstrates that there are a range of health benefits for switching from some feeding practices to breast milk supplemented with nonmilk liquids (table 3). There are only a few statistically significant effects increasing weight-for-age and reducing the prevalence of diarrhea, cough, and fever. These health benefits are only seen when switching from feeding practices that include solid foods. As was the case with switching to supplementation with milk liquids, other effects are positive or negative but are statistically insignificant due to high variability. Again it is of great interest to see the magnitude of these simulated effects.

Discussion

The results of our analysis simulating the effects of switching infant feeding practice to exclusive breastfeeding find positive health benefits for height, weight, and disease incidence. This general result is in keeping with the effects

Table 2. Simulated effects of switching to NEBF supplemented with milk liquids, age 0–6 months

Starting feeding practice	Length z score	Weight z score	Stunted
NEBF + solids	−0.021 (−0.123 to 0.081)	0.050 (−0.049 to 0.149)	−0.018 (−0.045 to 0.009)
NEBF + nonmilk liquids	−0.043 (−0.147 to 0.062)	−0.058 (−0.166 to 0.050)	0.006 (−0.022 to 0.034)
NEBF + infant formula	0.085 (−0.057 to 0.227)	−0.053 (−0.188 to 0.082)	−0.007 (−0.039 to 0.025)
NEBF + nonmilk liquids + milk liquids	−0.038 (−0.135 to 0.059)	0.043 (−0.050 to 0.137)	0.001 (−0.025 to 0.027)
NEBF + nonmilk liquids + solids	−0.059 (−0.185 to 0.066)	0.093 (−0.035 to 0.222)	−0.017 (−0.050 to 0.016)
NEBF + milk liquids + solids	−0.016 (−0.083 to 0.050)	0.152 (0.085 to 0.218)*	−0.023 (−0.039 to −0.006)*
NEBF + milk liquids + infant formula	0.090 (−0.031 to 0.210)	0.048 (−0.068 to 0.165)	−0.012 (−0.041 to 0.017)
NEBF + nonmilk liquids + infant formula	0.047 (−0.117 to 0.211)	−0.010 (−0.169 to 0.149)	−0.006 (−0.046 to 0.034)

Confidence intervals are presented in parentheses and based upon 1,000 bootstrapped replications of regression analysis. * $p < 0.05$.

Table 3. Simulated effects of switching to NEBF supplemented with nonmilk liquids, age 0–6 months

Starting feeding practice	Length z score	Weight z score	Stunted
NEBF + solids	0.022 (−0.095 to 0.138)	0.108 (−0.005 to 0.221)	−0.024 (−0.055 to 0.008)
NEBF + milk liquids	0.043 (−0.062 to 0.147)	0.058 (−0.050 to 0.166)	−0.006 (−0.034 to 0.022)
NEBF + infant formula	0.128 (−0.022 to 0.278)	0.005 (−0.143 to 0.153)	−0.013 (−0.050 to 0.025)
NEBF + nonmilk liquids + milk liquids	0.005 (−0.071 to 0.080)	0.101 (0.028 to 0.175)*	−0.005 (−0.024 to 0.015)
NEBF + nonmilk liquids + solids	−0.016 (−0.083 to 0.050)	0.152 (0.085 to 0.218)*	−0.023 (−0.039 to −0.006)*
NEBF + milk liquids + solids	0.026 (−0.096 to 0.148)	0.210 (0.084 to 0.335)*	−0.028 (−0.061 to 0.004)
NEBF + milk liquids + infant formula	0.133 (−0.022 to 0.287)	0.107 (−0.053 to 0.266)	−0.018 (−0.058 to 0.023)
NEBF + nonmilk liquids + infant formula	0.090 (−0.031 to 0.210)	0.048 (−0.068 to 0.165)	−0.012 (−0.041 to 0.017)

Confidence intervals are presented in parentheses and based upon 1,000 bootstrapped replications of regression analysis. * $p < 0.05$.

Wasted	Diarrhea	Fever	Cough
0.008 (−0.010 to 0.026)	−0.074 (−0.103 to −0.044)*	−0.053 (−0.088 to −0.017)*	−0.048 (−0.085 to −0.011)*
0.003 (−0.018 to 0.023)	−0.041 (−0.070 to −0.012)*	0.010 (−0.024 to 0.045)	0.023 (−0.015 to 0.061)
0.013 (−0.010 to 0.036)	−0.022 (−0.063 to 0.018)	0.021 (−0.027 to 0.068)	0.007 (−0.044 to 0.059)
−0.007 (−0.024 to 0.010)	−0.026 (−0.054 to 0.001)	−0.014 (−0.048 to 0.019)	0.003 (−0.033 to 0.039)
0.001 (−0.023 to 0.024)	−0.100 (−0.135 to −0.065)*	−0.067 (−0.107 to −0.027)*	−0.045 (−0.090 to 0.000)
−0.002 (−0.013 to 0.010)	−0.059 (−0.078 to −0.040)*	−0.077 (−0.099 to −0.055)*	−0.068 (−0.092 to −0.045)*
0.003 (−0.016 to 0.022)	−0.007 (−0.042 to 0.027)	−0.004 (−0.045 to 0.038)	−0.013 (−0.058 to 0.032)
0.006 (−0.023 to 0.035)	−0.048 (−0.096 to −0.001)*	0.006 (−0.050 to 0.062)	0.010 (−0.051 to 0.072)

Wasted	Diarrhea	Fever	Cough
0.005 (−0.015 to 0.026)	−0.033 (−0.067 to 0.001)	−0.063 (−0.105 to −0.020)*	−0.071 (−0.115 to −0.027)*
−0.003 (−0.023 to 0.018)	0.041 (0.012 to 0.070)*	−0.010 (−0.045 to 0.024)	−0.023 (−0.061 to 0.015)
0.010 (−0.013 to 0.033)	0.019 (−0.022 to 0.060)	0.011 (−0.039 to 0.061)	−0.016 (−0.070 to 0.037)
−0.010 (−0.024 to 0.005)	0.015 (−0.006 to −0.036)	−0.025 (−0.050 to 0.001)	−0.021 (−0.047 to 0.006)
−0.002 (−0.013 to 0.010)	−0.059 (−0.078 to −0.040)*	−0.077 (−0.099 to −0.055)*	−0.068 (−0.092 to −0.045)*
−0.004 (−0.028 to 0.019)	−0.018 (−0.053 to 0.017)	−0.087 (−0.130 to −0.045)*	−0.092 (−0.136 to −0.047)*
0.000 (−0.026 to 0.027)	0.034 (−0.009 to 0.076)	−0.014 (−0.066 to 0.038)	−0.037 (−0.092 to 0.019)
0.003 (−0.016 to 0.022)	−0.007 (−0.042 to 0.027)	−0.004 (−0.045 to 0.038)	−0.013 (−0.058 to 0.032)

seen elsewhere in the literature [1–9]. Our results provide additional information by quantifying the specific health effects of switching to exclusive breastfeeding. Additionally, we simulate the effects of switching between alternative feeding practices other than exclusive breastfeeding and quantify those effects.

Understanding the magnitude of the effect of feeding practices is essential for pediatricians as they seek to evaluate the average impact of feeding decisions and demonstrate the importance of feeding to their patients. While the effects we estimate here are simply the effect on average for a representative population, they can still be useful to individual cases. These results enable a pediatrician to say that on average an infant that is currently fed with breast milk and solid food, will reduce his fever incidence by 12.4% if he is switched to exclusive breastfeeding, 6.3% if he is switched to breast milk supplemented with nonmilk liquids, and 5.3% if he is switched to breast milk supplemented with milk liquids. Similarly, a pediatrician can say that an infant currently fed breast milk, milk liquids, and solid foods can increase his weight-for-age z score by 0.275 if he switches to exclusive breastfeeding, 0.152 if he switches to breast milk supplemented with milk liquids only, and 0.210 if he switches to breast milk supplemented with nonmilk liquids. These quantified estimates will help practitioners understand the average benefits of switching feeding practices and may help them convince patients of the importance of improving feeding practices. These are substantial health gains that may have long-lasting effects, so providing this quantified evidence to patients may help to convince them of the importance of improving infant feeding practices.

Quantifying the effect of infant feeding is also important for public health policymakers and practitioners. A significant component of improving infant feeding is through health education programs [13], so it is important to properly motivate support for these programs with quantified estimates of their effects. If the effect of programs is unknown, then it is much less likely to receive support or funding. A public health practitioner can point to these simulations to provide estimated impacts of a breastfeeding education program. Public health resources are frequently scarce, so policymakers want to guarantee that they are allocated properly. Cost-effectiveness analysis using simulated estimates like these is an important component of determining the best allocation of public health resources. Policymakers can simulate the specific health effect on their population of infants and use this to direct policy.

Importantly, our subsample testing indicates that the subsample used in this analysis is representative of overall feeding practices in the full DHS sample, suggesting that the simulated effects are generalizable across the full geography of the DHS. This generalizability makes a substantial contribution to the literature as most previous analyses have been emphasized as country or region specific.

This is important for pediatricians and public health practitioners that need to use estimated effects of infant feeding. Because this research is based on estimates from our past research, it has the same limitations as that work. These include the absence of longitudinal data and the problems that arise from causal inference and issues relating to recall data [12].

This research provides important information about the specific effects of feeding practices on infant health that have been lacking in the prior literature and are essential for decision-making by pediatricians and public health policymakers and practitioners. These quantified estimates of the effect of switching infant feeding practices can be used to motivate individual decisions about infant feeding and public health policy about infant feeding programs. Through these channels, they can hopefully play a role in improving infant health.

Disclosure Statement

Research was funded by Nestlé Nutrition Institute. The funding organization is an independent institute that is associated with a company that produces infant formula.

References

1 Lamberti LM, Fischer Walker CL, Noiman A, et al: Breastfeeding and the risk for diarrhea morbidity and mortality. BMC Public Health 2011;11(suppl 3):S15.

2 Lauer JA, Betrán AP, Barros AJ, de Onís M: Deaths and years of life lost due to suboptimal breast-feeding among children in the developing world: a global ecological risk assessment. Public Health Nutr 2006;9:673–685.

3 Simondon KB, Simondon F, Costes R, et al: Breast-feeding is associated with improved growth in length, but not weight, in rural Senegalese toddlers. Am J Clin Nutr 2001;73:959–967.

4 Saleemi MA, Ashraf RN, Mellander L, Zaman S: Determinants of stunting at 6, 12, 24 and 60 months and postnatal linear growth in Pakistani children. Acta Paediatr 2001;90:1304–1308.

5 Dewey KG, Cohen RJ, Brown KH, Rivera LL: Effects of exclusive breastfeeding for four versus six months on maternal nutritional status and infant motor development: results of two randomized trials in Honduras. J Nutr 2001;131:262–267.

6 Bhutta ZA, Ahmed T, Black RE, et al: What works? Interventions for maternal and child undernutrition and survival. Lancet 2008;371:417–440.

7 Kramer MS, Kakuma R: The optimal duration of exclusive breastfeeding: a systematic review. Adv Exp Med Biol 2004;554:63–77.

8 Bener A, Ehlayel MS, Alsowaidi S, Sabbah A: Role of breast feeding in primary prevention of asthma and allergic diseases in a traditional society. Eur Ann Allergy Clin Immunol 2007;39:337–343.

9 Bahl R, Frost C, Kirkwood BR, et al: Infant feeding patterns and risks of death and hospitalization in the first half of infancy: multicentre cohort study. Bull World Health Organ 2005;83:418–426.

10 World Health Organization: Global strategy for infant and young child feeding. Geneva, World Health Organization, 2003; http://whqlibdoc.who.int/publications/2003/9241562218.pdf.

11 Marriott BM, Campbell L, Hirsch E, Wilson D: Preliminary data from demographic and health surveys on infant feeding in 20 developing countries. J Nutr 2007;137:518S–523S.

12 Yarnoff B, Allaire B, Detzel P: Associations between infant feeding practices and length, weight, and disease in developing countries. Front Pediatr 2013;1:21.

13 Arusei RJ, Ettyang GA, Esamai F: Feeding patterns and growth of term infants in Eldoret, Kenya. Food Nutr Bull 2011;32:307–314.

Black RE, Singhal A, Uauy R (eds): International Nutrition: Achieving Millennium Goals and Beyond.
Nestlé Nutr Inst Workshop Ser, vol 78, pp 39–52, (DOI: 10.1159/000354935)
Nestec Ltd., Vevey/S. Karger AG., Basel, © 2014

Addressing the Double Burden of Malnutrition with a Common Agenda

Ricardo Uauy[a–c] · María Luisa Garmendia[a] · Camila Corvalán[a]

[a]Institute of Nutrition and Food Technology, University of Chile, and [b]Pediatric Department, Catholic University, Santiago de Chile, Chile; [c]London School of Hygiene and Tropical Medicine, London, UK

Abstract

Addressing *malnutrition in all its forms* represents an integrated agenda addressing the root causes of malnutrition at all stages of the life course. The issue is not about choosing between addressing undernutrition in the poor versus overnutrition in the affluent. We must recognize that the interventions required to address stunting are different from those needed to reduce underweight and wasting. In most developing regions, there is a coexistence between underweight and stunting in infants and children, while in the adult population it may be overweight and stunting. Malnutrition in all its forms refers to both underweight and overweight. Underweight is defined by a low weight-for-age, a child is underweight because of wasting (low weight-for-height) or stunting (low length-for-age). Stunting refers to low height-for-age independent of their weight-for-age, some stunted children may have excess weight for their stature length. Overweight is excess weight-for-length/-height or high-BMI-for-age. The prevention of nutrition-related chronic diseases is a life-long process that starts in fetal life and continues throughout infancy and later stages of life. It requires promoting healthy diets and active living at each stage. The agenda requires that we tackle malnutrition in all its forms.

© 2014 Nestec Ltd., Vevey/S. Karger AG, Basel

Introduction

The burden of malnutrition and related death, disease and disability has multiple dimensions in the developing as well as in the industrialized regions of the world that are often ignored by experts and laypersons alike. The reality of nutritional problems today, in most of the world is somewhat of a paradox. Presently, poor countries in which most of the undernutrition burden is concentrated are also suffering rising prevalence of obesity and related noncommunicable disease (NCD) burden [1]. The same policies and programs that successfully served to prevent and control malnutrition in times of slow economic growth or during economic depression are now potentially contributing to the NCD epidemic in developing countries. These policies in most developing and transitional countries have included securing access to food energy sources (mostly cereals, fats and oils) in support of food security. Subsidizing the price of sugar, cereals (wheat, rice, bread), other refined starches, vegetable oil (soy, rapeseed and corn) and in some cases alcohol and animal fat has contributed to generating an obesogenic environment. As malnutrition and infections retreat, progressive inactivity due to changes in the nature of physical work related to productive activities and rural-urban migration serve to reduce energy expenditure during both work and leisure time. This undoubtedly has contributed to fuel the progressive epidemic rise in noncommunicable chronic diseases in developing and transitional countries [2]. International agencies, NGOs and academics dealing with malnutrition were initially reluctant to acknowledge that developing countries were facing a 'double burden of disease'. However, the extent of NCD epidemic and a better understanding of causes and consequences has led to a present consensus that malnutrition has to be addressed considering the consequences of both deficit and excess energy. The present aim is to continue efforts to lower undernutrition without increasing obesity and the associated NCDs.

The Double Burden of Malnutrition

Undernutrition is no longer the dominant form of human malnutrition globally; coexistence of the dual expressions of under- and overnutrition can be exemplified globally at all levels. In 2011, the estimated number of people worldwide suffering from overweight [with a body mass index (BMI) >25] exceeded those with underweight (<2 standard deviations (SD) below the WHO reference median). Recent estimates indicate that over a billion individuals are overweight or obese, and a slightly lower number are underweight [3]. However, the demographic distribution is age specific, with more obesity in adults in developed countries and more malnutrition in children in developing countries. Further disaggregation reveals just how closely the two conditions coexist. Figure 1 presents the proportion of deaths and disability-adjusted life years (DALYs) lost from conditions of communicable, noncommunicable diseases and injuries. For both high- and middle-income countries, NCDs represent the main causes of

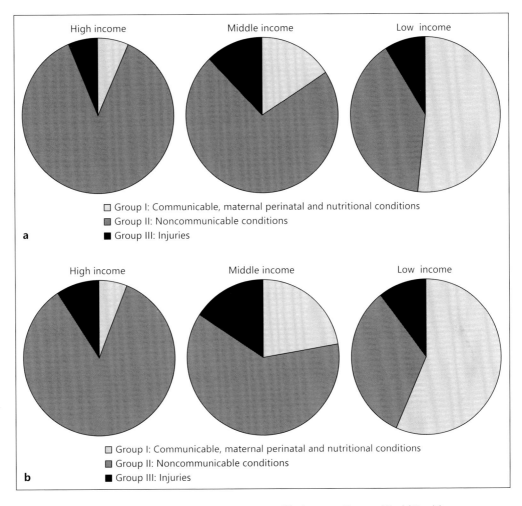

Fig. 1. a Deaths by disease category, countries grouped by income. Source: World Health Organization [24]. **b** DALYs by disease category, countries grouped by income. Source: WHO [24].

death and disability, while in low-income countries infectious disease remains as the main cause of death. Table 1 shows the changes in the ranking of the top ten nutrition-related risks that accounted for loss of healthy life years and of lives over the past 2 decades. Table 2 provides a further breakdown of the causes of death and disability globally and disaggregated by four levels of income.

Generating common policies and intervention to address the double burden is particularly important in those nations and regions in which one sees appreciable loss of DALYs from both conditions, such as Northern Africa and Middle East, most of South, Southeast and East Asia, Central America and the Andean region [4].

Table 1. Nutrition-based risk factors for global burden of disease (1990–2010)

	DALYs		Deaths	
	1990	2010	1990	2010
Childhood underweight	1	8	7	16
Suboptimal breastfeeding	5	14	14	20
Iron deficiency	11	13	29	33
Vitamin A deficiency	17	29	23	32
Zinc deficiency	19	31	26	37
High blood pressure	4	1	1	1
Low fruit	8	5	4	3
High sodium	12	11	8	10
High BMI	10	6	10	7
High fasting plasma glucose	9	7	9	6

Source: Global Burden of Disease Study 2010.

The presence of a double burden within the same nation is the next level of aggregation; the recent 2013 WHO statistics provides a perspective on how under- and overnutrition operate within the same regions, specifically in reference to children <5 years of age. Figure 2 illustrates the percentage of children in different world regions with height-for-age z scores either below (stunting) or above (overweight) 2 SD of the international reference median; the burden is dual on a population basis where the prevalence in both directions exceeds >2.5% on the horizontal axis. Although stunting continues to be the most prevalent nutritional problem in all regions except Europe, overweight exceeds 5% in most regions. Within the same community or even within a given household, the presence of both over- and undernutrition takes on some interesting dimensions. Caballero [5] has further scrutinized the phenomenon of persons with high and low bodyweights living within the same household. The interpretation of this phenomenon may be in part explained by low prevalence of one or the other condition limiting the opportunity to define causal pathways. However, as incomes rise, one can observe the occurrence of extremes in body composition and nutritional status existing within the same family unit; commonly stunted children and obese mothers.

Finally, within a given individual, namely a malnourished young child, there can be a quick transition, over a matter of several weeks or a few months, from being wasted (underweight-for-height) to being overweight or even obese while remaining stunted (excess weight-for-height); moreover, in many cases these children remain chronically stunted (low height-for-age), making

Table 2. Causes of death and disability globally and disaggregated by four levels of income

a Population attributable fraction for mortality (%) by risk factor, and country income group, estimates for 2004

Cause	World	High income	Upper middle income	Lower middle income	Low income
Childhood and maternal undernutrition					
Underweight	3.8	0.0	0.2	0.9	7.8
Iron deficiency	0.5	0.1	0.2	0.2	0.8
Vitamin A deficiency	1.1	0.0	0.1	0.4	2.2
Zinc deficiency	0.7	0.0	0.1	0.2	1.5
Suboptimal breastfeeding	2.1	0.1	0.5	1.3	3.7
Other nutrition-related risk factors and physical activity					
High blood pressure	12.8	16.8	22.8	15.5	7.5
High cholesterol	4.5	5.8	8.5	4.2	3.4
High blood glucose	5.8	7.0	8.1	5.8	4.9
Overweight and obesity	4.8	8.4	11.7	5.3	1.9
Low fruit and vegetable intake	2.8	2.5	4.8	3.6	2.0
Physical inactivity	5.5	7.7	9.5	5.7	3.8
Addictive substances					
Tobacco use	8.7	17.9	13.4	10.0	3.9
Alcohol use	3.8	1.6	9.4	5.5	2.2
Illicit drug use	0.4	0.4	0.5	0.4	0.4
Sexual and reproductive health					
Unsafe sex	4.0	0.5	6.6	1.2	6.6
Unmet contraceptive need	0.3	0.0	0.0	0.1	0.5
Environmental risks					
Unsafe water, sanitation, hygiene	3.2	0.1	0.5	1.4	6.1
Urban outdoor air pollution	2.0	2.5	2.4	2.9	1.0
Indoor smoke from solid fuels	3.3	0.0	0.2	3.6	4.8
Lead exposure	0.2	0.0	0.2	0.3	0.3
Global climate change	0.2	0.0	0.0	0.1	0.5
Occupational risks	1.7	1.1	1.4	2.6	1.3
Other selected risks					
Unsafe health care injections	0.8	2.8	0.3	1.3	0.6
Child sexual abuse	0.1	0.1	0.1	0.1	0.2

Source: WHO. Health Statistics and health information systems. Risk factors estimates for 2004.

them more vulnerable in an urban setting to obesity and diabetes, both of which are linked to excess body fat resulting from sedentary lifestyles and consumption of high-energy-density diets. In fact, the model of the malnourished child during recovery serves to illustrate many of the features of the nutrition transition; it is in fact the rapid shift in diet from low- to high-energy-density food, as well as a progressively sedentary lifestyle that moves stunted popula-

Table 2. Causes of death and disability globally and disaggregated by four levels of income

b Population attributable fraction for DALYs (%) by risk factor and country income group, estimates for 2004

Cause	World	High income	Upper middle income	Lower middle income	Low income
Childhood and maternal undernutrition					
Underweight	5.9	0.1	0.7	1.7	9.9
Iron deficiency	1.3	0.5	0.7	1.1	1.6
Vitamin A deficiency	1.4	0.0	0.2	0.5	2.4
Zinc deficiency	1.0	0.0	0.1	0.3	1.7
Suboptimal breastfeeding	2.9	0.3	0.9	1.9	4.1
Other nutrition-related risk factors and physical activity					
High blood pressure	3.7	6.1	8.2	4.7	2.2
High cholesterol	1.9	3.4	4.3	2.0	1.4
High blood glucose	2.7	4.9	4.4	3.1	1.9
Overweight and obesity	2.3	6.5	6.7	2.8	0.8
Low fruit and vegetable intake	1.0	1.3	2.1	1.4	0.7
Physical inactivity	2.1	4.1	4.2	2.4	1.3
Addictive substances					
Tobacco use	3.7	10.7	8.3	4.6	1.5
Alcohol use	4.5	6.7	11.5	6.5	2.1
Illicit drug use	0.9	2.1	1.3	1.0	0.6
Sexual and reproductive health					
Unsafe sex	4.6	0.9	8.9	1.5	6.2
Unmet contraceptive need	0.8	0.0	0.3	0.4	1.1
Environmental risks					
Unsafe water, sanitation, hygiene	4.2	0.3	0.9	2.2	6.3
Urban outdoor air pollution	0.6	0.8	0.8	0.8	0.3
Indoor smoke from solid fuels	2.7	0.0	0.2	1.6	4.0
Lead exposure	0.6	0.1	0.4	0.7	0.6
Global climate change	0.4	0.0	0.0	0.1	0.6
Occupational risks	1.7	1.5	1.7	2.5	1.2
Other selected risks					
Unsafe health care injections	0.5	1.8	0.2	0.7	0.4
Child sexual abuse	0.6	0.7	0.5	0.6	0.6

Source: WHO. Health Statistics and health information systems. Risk factors estimates for 2004.

tions from underweight to overweight and obesity [6]. Rapid shifts in weight (catch-up) without concurrent gains in height are now recognized as particularly increasing the risk of later diabetes, central obesity and cardiovascular diseases [6]. HIV/AIDS also serves as an example of the dual burden in a single disease entity. In the fully expressed immunodeficiency state, the wasting processes induced by the retrovirus infection itself or in combination

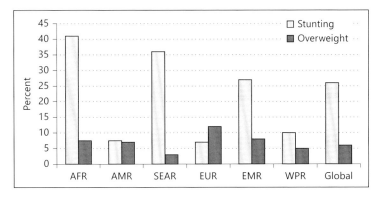

Fig. 2. Prevalence of stunting and overweight in children aged <5 years by WHO region, 2011. AFR = WHO African region; AMR = WHO region of the Americas; SEAR = WHO South-East Asia region; EUR = WHO European region; EMR = WHO Mediterranean region; WPR = WHO Western Pacific region. Source: WHO [25].

with opportunistic infections of the host lead to the so called 'slim disease'. However, if adequately treated, HIV may also progress to a chronic condition associated with vascular disease (atherosclerosis) induced by alterations of lipid and glucose metabolism as well as hypertension and renal damage [7, 8].

Two Sides of the Coin in the Developmental Origins of Health

A complex and intriguing – yet compelling – relationship has been revealed between the processes of undernutrition and poor growth in early life (fetal and infancy) and obesity with its associated consequences on metabolic and cancer in adult life [9, 10]. Prof. David Barker, the unquestionable pioneer in the area of epidemiology of early origins of adult disease [11], coined the term, 'early life programming' based on a persistence of a nutrient-conserving metabolic pattern throughout the lifespan. Gluckman et al. [12] have given a less pathocentric, and more adaptive, connotation to the relationship of early low growth, metabolic imprinting, and vulnerability to chronic disease. Thus, the metabolic patterning is shaped by afferent signals to the fetus from the maternal environment. If a hostile and nutrient-scarce environment is perceived, nutrient-conserving mechanisms are put in place; if nutrient abundance is sensed, normal nutrient disposal is programmed. Concordance between the intrauterine choice and the external reality in later life represents an adaptive match. Discordance, however, leads to an adverse adaptation leading to increased risk of either undernutrition or noncommunicable illnesses, depending on the direction of the mismatch. In the case of developing countries, fetal and infant undernutrition is still very prevalent while obesogenic environments are becoming progressively more common. The mismatch will result in an increased predisposition to obesity and related NCDs. On the nutrient excess side, macrosomia (birthweight >4,000 g or alternatively ≥+2 SD of the bodyweight distribution) corresponds to the alternate maladaptive nutritional condition in fetal life. All share the consequences of adverse for long-term health prognosis. Excessive intrauterine growth, mainly fat tissue accumulation but also glycogen loading of liver and muscle, is due to excess glucose and higher insulin levels during the last trimester of pregnancy as a result of gestational hyperglycemia in the mother and the corresponding fetal hyperinsulinemia [13].

Cohort studies of macrosomic infants have shown that high birthweight and overweight in infancy are risk factors for obesity and diabetes in later life [14]. Independent of the order of the sequence, from underweight to overweight (in the case of the growth-restricted infant) or from overweight to overweight (in the case of the macrosomic infant), the consequence of the altered fetal metabolic-nutritional state in later life (adolescence and adulthood) is an increased burden of chronic disease compromising even further societies that are barely coping with the economic costs of undernutrition.

The Life Course Approach to Nutrition

Nutrition should be seen as a continuous process from the womb to the tomb. The so-called nutrition-infection complex determines, in large part, how children grow and develop mentally, while diet-physical activity interactions greatly affect what diseases we will most likely suffer from during our lifespan and, finally, how we will age and die. As we have discussed earlier in this chapter, the preconceptional maternal nutritional status influences the conceptus, determining fetal and infant nutrition and growth. A wide range of factors operate within each particular stage and interact with genetic constitution to influence the nutritional status of the individual in that particular phase of life, but also cumulatively in the later stages of the lifespan. The practical implications are that we need a better definition of 'malnutrition' in order to guide our situational analysis leading to appropriately designed 'evidence-based interventions' that consider the life course approach as a template to identify the most cost-effective interventions to reduce morbidity and health care costs across all stages of the lifespan. Our ultimate goal should be what Fries [15] has termed the 'compression of morbidity', meaning that we live lives free of the disabilities related to acute and chronic illnesses and impaired function and extend our healthy life years towards the upper limits of the human lifespan, for now circa 105 years.

Double Burden of Malnutrition on the International Political Agenda

Monitoring the content of the newsletter published by the UN-SCN (Standing Committee on Nutrition) which in the past decades served to harmonize/coordinate the actions taken by the UN system (WHO/FAO/WFP/UNICEF/WB/UNU/UNESCO/UNHCR) and bilateral agencies in the area of food and nutrition, one can verify a major shift in the balance of themes for discussion and proposal for actions related to the double burden (under and over nutrition) starting in 1980. The debate came to a climax in 1998, at its 25th Annual Session in Oslo and in 1999 at its 26th Annual Session in Geneva in which SCN discussed the Report of the Commission on the Nutrition Challenges of the Twenty-First Century: What Role for the United Nations? This report commission by the SCN itself to an independent group of outside experts in food, agriculture, health, and economic development including members of the SCN's own AGN (advisory group on nutrition) challenged the UN system to acknowledge the existence of the double burden on malnutrition with a life course perspective. Two of the eight main challenges posed and debated by the UN-SCN in 2000 addressed the dual nature of global nutrition problems. The discussions that took place in Geneva in 1999 were followed by the adoption of 'Nutrition throughout the Life Cycle' as the theme for the 4th World Nutrition Report. This report highlighted the emergence of the double burden, stating that: 'Among adults, both under- and over-nutrition are present in many countries in the developing world. While underweight is especially common among women in South Central Asia, both underweight and overweight is seen in African women. In the Caribbean and Latin America, overweight affects up to one in four women in all countries surveyed, except in Haiti'. Some of the SCN members, at the time, had difficulty dealing with the concept of a double burden of malnutrition; several agencies chose to disassociate themselves from the main conclusions and recommendations of this report. The report also recommended the use of the term 'malnutrition in all its forms' to encompass all nutritional problems, addressing them in with integrated approaches rather than continuing to pursue the single nutrient 'magic bullet' interventions which prevail to present times. The report recommended abandoning the sterile debate on which single nutrient should take precedence over others and recommended a common definition adopting the term malnutrition in all its forms which leads to policies that combine approaches and integrate policies and programs.

That same year 2000, Gro Harlem Brundtland became the Director-General of WHO and propelled nutrition-related chronic diseases to the top of the agenda, because of its contribution to the challenges of the global burden of death and disability. In 2002, WHO lead by Brundtland after recruiting two able collaborators in the theme, Derek Yach and Pekka Puska convened an expert group to develop a technical report (WHO TRS-916 published in 2003). A year later in 2004 a global strategy to address diet and physical activity prevention of chronic disease was formulated and presented to the WHO general assembly and approved in 2004 [16]. The report acknowledged that NCDs were and remain the greatest cause of global mortality with 29 million deaths annually due to cardiovascular disease, cancer, chronic respiratory disease and diabetes. It noted that the UN system public health responses by professional groups and governments remain inadequate even to date commenting that: 'Reasons for this include that up to date evidence related to the nature of the burden of chronic diseases is not in the hands of decision makers and strong beliefs persist that chronic diseases afflict only the affluent and the elderly, that they arise solely from freely ado risks, and that their control is ineffective and too expensive and should wait until infectious diseases are addressed'. A body of evidence has demonstrated that, unfortunately, once again the poor are most affected by this new epidemic. The various linkages in poverty/low income and body composition are well illustrated by the analysis of the Latin American situation conducted by Peña and Bacallao [17] and a series of national nutrition surveys conducted in Brazil over decades. Initially, the poor had normal or low bodyweights and the middle class had the greater prevalence of overweight. Over time, however, the situation reversed; by the late 1990s, Brazilian elite had recovered normal body composition, while the poor were manifesting overweight and obesity [18]. It seems that the affluent have better access to education and exhibit health-seeking behaviors. The rich were able to adopt better quality diets and live more actively while the urban poor, constrained by low-quality food, crowded housing and newly acquired sedentary lifestyle suffer the consequences to a greater extent.

Furthermore, as illustrated by the experience in Chile as in most of Latin America to date, the nutrition intervention programs destined for the undernourished fail to recognize that most underweight children are also stunted. In the case of Chile, height was not systematically measured until 1992, so that those with apparent normal weight-for-age were commonly of low height, thus were overweight or obese. Providing excess energy to promote weight gain was clearly not the answer. Thus, we need to particularly focus on obesity prevention when feeding stunted populations [19]. The compendium of chapters collected and edited by Caballero and Popkin in 2002, Nutrition Transition: Diet and Disease in Developing Countries, adds layer upon layer of additional evidence on the associations, at times causal, between being of lower social level, having fewer economic resources and suffering from overweight, obesity and chronic diseases [20]. Finally, despite the initial difficulties in recognizing the dual nature (under-over) of the prevailing forms of malnutrition, the topic was placed on the agenda of the SCN. In fact, the 33rd Annual Session symposium (March 2006) was a landmark SCN session calling for 'Tackling the Double Burden of Malnutrition with a Common Agenda' and challenging the member countries to examine what needs to be done and what can be done at national, regional and international levels.

Need for a Common Operational Definition of Malnutrition

In order to tackle malnutrition in all its forms with a common agenda, it is necessary to agree on how to define malnutrition. The definition should be clear, easy to understand not only by experts but also more importantly by key stakeholders, policy-makers, politicians and the public at large. A commonly accepted definition is pivotal in tackling malnutrition in all its forms with a unified approach. We cannot afford to postpone efforts to prevent premature death of adults from nutrition-related chronic disease based on the argument that we need to first concentrate on undernutrition to avoid death in young children as the single priority. Projected estimates of the rise in obesity and NCD epidemic are striking; they show that if no actions are taken to control them, in less than two decades NCDs will more than double in low- and middle-income countries, imposing an unbearable burden for the developing economies of these countries. Moreover, as we present in this review, deficit and excess are intertwined at different levels; thus, the consequences of what we do or fail to do in either will affect society in multiple ways. The answer, when allocating resources, is not choosing between these two but rather addressing them jointly with an integrated approach.

A proposal presented at the SCN's 33rd Annual Session considered the following definition of terms to help advance in forging a common agenda: Malnutrition in all its forms includes: underweight, wasting, stunting and overweight, as well as micronutrient deficiencies and nutrition-related chronic diseases. Underweight was defined by a low weight-for-age; a child may be underweight because she or he is wasted (low weight-for-height) or is stunted (low height-for-age), or both. Wasting and stunting should be considered separately since they require different approaches to their treatment and control. Low birthweight is defined as being underweight at the time of birth (below 2,500 g), whereas the growth-restricted newborn is one that has low birthweight for the corresponding gestational age (based on an accepted standard, as presently being developed by the INTERGROWTH study). Acute wasting is an important form of malnutrition, especially within the context of emergencies and child survival since it has a direct impact on resistance to infection. To attain the respective MDGs on child hunger and mortality necessitates effective treatment and control of acute wasting. Stunting refers to low height-for-age, independent of weight-for-age; in fact, some stunted children may have normal or even excess weight-for-height. Overweight refers to excess weight for one's length or stature, measured as weight-for-height or BMI centile for age (BMI is kg/m^2), depending on cutoffs for overweight or obesity categories. Micronutrient deficiencies are due to poor quality of diets and nutrient wasting caused by infection and chronic inflammation; deficiencies can be single or affecting multiple micronutrients and should be categorized according to the respective micronutrient involved. Nutrition-related chronic diseases are chronic diseases common in adults, related to diet and physical activity (e.g. cardiovascular diseases, obesity/diabetes, some forms of cancer and osteoporosis).

There is also a need to update the indicators we use to monitor nutritional progress. If we continue to assess nutrition based on weight-for-age alone, and not use the combination of weight-for-height and height-for-age indices, we will be unable to recognize and properly address stunting, presently the most frequent alteration of growth. Stunting provides a cumulative record of past and present conditions restricting linear growth. In the short term, stunting affects both mortality and morbidity particularly due to infectious diseases such as diarrhea, measles, pneumonia, and malaria; in the long term, it is also related to increased obesity and risk for metabolic disease such as diabetes and hyperlipidemia [21, 22]. Thus, stunting prevention is key to effectively address malnutrition in all its forms not only for this but also for future generations.

Health outcomes also have to be reexamined with a common perspective. We should continue using short-term outcomes such as survival or acute morbidity but complement them with indicators of long-term outcomes. There is now increasing evidence that diet and physical activity behaviors as well as metabolic/hormonal responses are shaped early on in life and track thereafter. Interventions required to address stunting are different from those needed to reduce underweight and wasting. Actions have to focus more on diet quality than on diet quantity; food supplements should secure energy but also be composed of the right fat, carbohydrate and protein quality. Actions should be aimed at pregnant women and infants; the existence of other 'critical/sensitive' periods for preventive interventions should be explored. Current interventions to prevent stunting account for only 36% of the cases of stunting at 36 months [23]; current obesity- and NCD-preventive actions also show limited success. In order to improve the results of preventive action, diet-physical activity-infection interactions should be revisited considering a life course approach. We clearly need new ideas leading to novel and more effective actions; research on how to best deliver these actions at the population level should also be optimized. We need to move from efficacy to true effectiveness studies under real-world conditions; the search for cost-effective solutions should be the goal. Finally, structural level actions such as empowering women, improving sanitation levels, access to basic health and education for all are key components that can accelerate progress.

Disclosure Statement

Dr. Uauy is the president of the Nevin Scrimshaw International Nutrition Foundation. His recent and present research activities have been funded primarily by Fondecyt Chile (National Science and Technology Fund), the Wellcome Trust UK, the World Cancer Research Fund, and the US National Institutes of Health. He has provided over the past 20 years technical advice in areas of his competence to International UN and non UN related organizations (WHO/FAO/UNICEF/WFP/UN-SCN). He does not own personal stock except for investment funds related to his pension that are not under his direct control. Dr. Uauy is a member of national (Chile) and regional (Americas region) technical advisory committees related to areas of his technical competence (food/nutrition/ health). He does not hold or have pending patent applications related or unrelated to his research activities. He receives funds from copyrights related to books that he has authored, and he serves as Associate Editor of the American Journal of Clinical Nutrition the International Journal of Obesity and of the Journal of Pediatric Gastroenterology and Nutrition.

References

1 World Health Organization: Global Health Risks: Mortality and burden of disease attributable to selected major risks. Geneva, World Health Organization, 2009.

2 Miranda JJ, Kinra S, Casas JP, et al: Non-communicable diseases in low- and middle-income countries: context, determinants and health policy. Trop Med Int Health 2008;13: 1225–1234.

3 World Health Organization Media Centre: Obesity and overweight, fact sheet No 311. Geneva, World Health Organization, 2012.

4 Murray CJ, Vos T, Lozano R, et al: Disability-adjusted life years (DALYs) for 291 diseases and injuries in 21 regions, 1990–2010: a systematic analysis for the Global Burden of Disease Study 2010. Lancet 2012;380:2197–2223.

5 Caballero B: A nutrition paradox – underweight and obesity in developing countries. N Engl J Med 2005;352:1514–1516.

6 Uauy R, Alvear J: Effects of protein energy interactions on growth; in Nevin S Scrimshaw, Beat Schürch (eds): Protein-Energy Interactions. Lausanne, UN ACC-Subcommittee on Nutrition, 1992.

7 Mooser V, Carr A: Antiretroviral therapy-associated hyperlipidaemia in HIV disease. Curr Opin Lipidol 2001;12:313–319.

8 Roling J, Schmid H, Fischereder M, et al: HIV-associated renal diseases and highly active antiretroviral therapy-induced nephropathy. Clin Infect Dis 2006;42:1488–1495.

9 McMillen IC, Robinson JS: Developmental origins of the metabolic syndrome: prediction, plasticity, and programming. Physiol Rev 2005;85:571–633.

10 Uauy R, Solomons N: Diet, nutrition, and the life-course approach to cancer prevention. J Nutr 2005;135(suppl 12):2934S–2945S.

11 Barker D: Mothers, Babies, and Health in Later Life, ed 2. Edinburg, Elsevier Health Sciences, 1988.

12 Gluckman PD, Cutfield W, Hofman P, Hanson MA: The fetal, neonatal, and infant environments-the long-term consequences for disease risk. Early Hum Dev 2005;81:51–59.

13 Leguizamon G, von Stecher F: Third trimester glycemic profiles and fetal growth. Curr Diab Rep 2003;3:323–326.

14 Das UG, Sysyn GD: Abnormal fetal growth: intrauterine growth retardation, small for gestational age, large for gestational age. Pediatr Clin North Am 2004;51:639–654, viii.

15 Fries JF: Measuring and monitoring success in compressing morbidity. Ann Intern Med 2003;139:455–459.

16 Yach D, Hawkes C, Gould CL, Hofman KJ: The global burden of chronic diseases: overcoming impediments to prevention and control. JAMA 2004;291:2616–2622.

17 Peña M, Bacallao J (eds): Obesity and Poverty: A New Public Health Challenge . Pan American Health Organization (PAHO), Washington DC, 2000.

18 Monteiro CA, D'A Benicio MH, Conde WL, Popkin BM: Shifting obesity trends in Brazil. Eur J Clin Nutr 2000;54:342–346.

19 Uauy R, Kain J: The epidemiological transition: need to incorporate obesity prevention into nutrition programmes. Public Health Nutr 2002;5:223–229.

20 Caballero B, Popkin BM (eds): The Nutrition Transition: Diet and Disease in the Developing World. Food Science and Technology International Series. London, Academic Press, 2002.

21 Hoffman DJ, Sawaya AL, Verreschi I, et al: Why are nutritionally stunted children at increased risk of obesity? Studies of metabolic rate and fat oxidation in shantytown children from Sao Paulo, Brazil. Am J Clin Nutr 2000; 72:702–707.

22 Gonzalez-Barranco J, Ríos-Torres JM, Castillo-Martínez L, et al: Effect of malnutrition during the first year of life on adult plasma insulin and glucose tolerance. Metabolism 2003;52:1005–1011.

23 Bhutta ZA, Ahmed T, Black RE, et al: What works? Interventions for maternal and child undernutrition and survival. Lancet 2008; 371:417–440.

24 World Health Organization: The global burden of disease: 2004 update. Geneva, World Health Organization, 2008.

25 World Health Organization: World Health Statistics 2013. Geneva, World Health Organization, 2013.

Black RE, Singhal A, Uauy R (eds): International Nutrition: Achieving Millennium Goals and Beyond.
Nestlé Nutr Inst Workshop Ser, vol 78, pp 53–58, (DOI: 10.1159/000354938)
Nestec Ltd., Vevey/S. Karger AG., Basel, © 2014

Summary on World Nutrition Situation

Jorge Jimenez presented the model successfully applied in Chile over the past century in order to address health and malnutrition. A clear focus on mother and child social protection was considered a key step in defining successful public health policies around the world. Most of the basic strategies are known and have been described, and their efficacy and cost-effectiveness have been demonstrated several times in different settings in the last 100 years. However, taking knowledge to action and moving from knowledge to public impact requires different approaches. Commonly, there is a major gap, which needs mending by other policy options. Beyond technical considerations, conviction, commitment and mystique were in his view and experience the key critical factors for success. The other key issue is close relation between academia, policy making, regular politics and public opinion. He recalled personal experience and reviewed mother and child health policies in the last 50 or more years in Chile, the country where he has played a major role in shaping policies. The first registered event on child health policy in Chile was in 1912. Many interventions with progressive coverage were implemented during decades of improvement in health care policies. The early emphasis in nutrition was quite clear from the start. With the consolidation of a National Health Service in the 1950s, Chile established a mother and child health policy based on the typical pillars of action: antenatal care, professional attention of deliveries, family planning, nutrition programs, well baby clinics, immunizations, respiratory and gastrointestinal infection therapies and water and sanitation projects in poor communities. The basic ideas were developed and tested by a group of socially sensitive academics from Universidad de Chile, who went to the community, studied the sociomedical conditions, proposed and essayed their interventions (1955–1960) and after having the conviction, 'took power' by accessing key posts in the NHS (1960–

1965). Impact was visible by the late 1970s, ironically during a period of military dictatorship, neoliberal reforms to the economy and deep recessions. The social-medical model for child survival proved to be stronger than most would have predicted; despite the tensions, programs continued to be implemented and advanced leading to a virtual eradication of malnutrition before 2000, and Chile was able to report success in meeting the UNICEF World Summit for Children Goals.

Benjamin Yarnoff considered the effect of infant feeding practices on height, weight, and disease in developing countries. Examining infant health in developing countries, focusing solely on breastfeeding or exclusive breastfeeding ignores the complexity of infant feeding and fails to acknowledge the multiple interactions that play important roles. Infants in developing countries receive a wide range of foods even when apparently are predominantly breastfed. For example, 22% of mothers in a survey of 20 developing countries feed their infants a range of solid foods before 6 months of age. The health benefits of exclusive breastfeeding are well known, but the relative detrimental effects of other foods on infant health are unknown. Because of the range of infant feeding practices in developing countries, understanding the health effects of these diverse feeding practices is essential for public health. The study conducted by *Benjamin Yarnoff* is one of the first to systematically examine the effect of a range of infant feeding practices on infant health for a large sample. He used data from the Demographic Health Survey from 20 developing countries over multiple years to examine the effect of six types of feeding (exclusive breastfeeding, nonexclusive breastfeeding, infant formula, milk liquids, non-milk liquids, and solid foods) on five health outcomes (height-for-age z score, weight-for-height z score, diarrhea, fever, and cough) for infants in two age groups (less than 6 months and 6 months to 1 year). Unlike previous work, he controlled for most potentially confounding factors. Consistent with previous studies, he finds that breastfeeding is beneficial for infant health and provides specific micro-level estimates of breastfeeding effects. He reports that the while all other types of feeding are inferior to breastfeeding, some have more harmful effects on infant health than others. This underscores the importance of differentiating between feeding types for public health programs seeking to improve infant health in developing countries.

Ricardo Uauy presented the multiple dimensions of the burden of malnutrition and related death, disease and disability affecting the developing as well as industrialized regions of the world. The reality of nutritional problems today, in most of the world is somewhat of a paradox. Presently, poor countries in which most of the undernutrition burden is concentrated are also suffering rising prevalence of obesity and related noncommunicable disease (NCD) burden. The same policies and programs that successfully served to prevent and control malnutrition in times of slow economic growth or during economic depression are now potentially contributing to the NCD epidemic in developing countries. These policies in most developing and transitional countries have included securing access to food energy sources (mostly cereals, fats and oils) in support of food security. Subsidizing the price of sugar, cereals (wheat, rice and bread) and other refined starches, vegetable oil (soy, rapeseed and corn) and in some cases alcohol and animal fat has contributed to generating an obesogenic environment. As malnutrition and infections retreat, progressive inactivity due to changes in the nature of physical work related to productive activities and rural-urban migration serve to reduce energy expenditure both during work and leisure time. This undoubtedly has contributed to fuelling the progressive epidemic rise in noncommunicable chronic diseases in developing and transitional countries. International agencies, NGOs and academics dealing with malnutrition were initially reluctant to acknowledge that developing countries were facing a 'double burden of disease'. However, the extent of NCD epidemic and a better understanding of causes and consequences has led to a present consensus that malnutrition has to be addressed considering the consequences of both deficit and excess energy. The present aim is to continue efforts to lower undernutrition without increasing obesity and the associated NCDs.

Andrew Dorward examined how agricultural interventions can contribute in improving nutrition health and achieving the MDGs in least developed countries. The strong conceptual linkages between agricultural development and nutrition improvements were discussed presenting three main pathways that may be used to characterize these linkages. The overall national development efforts, the promotion of self-sufficiency by producing one's own food and finally the market pathways is an alternate way to secure food for all; provided people's income is compatible with this goal. Evidence on the efficacy of these various pathways was presented, results are mixed, in some cases there are strong positive effects while in other the effects may be somewhat negative and in a third case there may only be weak impacts. The findings reflect both the importance of agriculture for nutrition and its dependence on contextual factors. They are also the result of insufficient high-quality empirical research investigating these linkages. The most effective 'pathways' and interventions linking agricultural change to improved nutritional outcomes change with economic growth and development, with declining importance of the development and own-production pathways and increasing importance of the market pathway. Substantial challenges in operationalizing agricultural-nutrition linkages need to be overcome to better exploit potential opportunities. *Andrew Dorward* drew attention to the fact that most recent information on progress and likely achievement or non-achievement of MDG targets is found in the UN. Substantial gains have been made in some regions (notably Western Asia, Eastern Asia, Caucasus and Central Asia and Latin America and the Caribbean, and to a lesser extent in North Africa and South Eastern Asia). However, progress has been slower in Sub-Saharan Africa and South Asia, and the overall target of halving the prevalence of undernourishment is unlikely to be met by 2015.

As with other MDG targets, there are wide variations between regions as regards changes in prevalence and numbers of undernourished people. FAO and WFP estimate that absolute numbers of undernourished people have been falling in Asia and in the Latin America-Caribbean areas, with falls in prevalence on track to meet the MDG target. In both Near East/North Africa and Sub-Saharan Africa, however, absolute numbers of undernourished people have been rising, with lower falls in prevalence in Sub-Saharan Africa, but actual increases in prevalence in Near East and North Africa – although this is from a much lower 1990–1992 starting point than the other regions (7% as compared with 15% in Latin America-Caribbean, 25% in Asia and 35% in Sub-Saharan Africa). There has been a remarkable fall in prevalence in South Eastern Asia from 30 to 11% from 1990–1992 to 2010, with a slightly lower but still remarkable fall in Eastern Asia from 21 to 12% over the same period. South Asia achieved a lower fall in prevalence, however, which if continued will not be enough to achieve the target. Prevalence in Western Asia increased.

There is a growing recognition that food availability is a necessary but insufficient condition for food security – access is also necessary through entitlements (allowing local unavailability to be overcome by purchases), and once accessed, food needs to be utilized. Utilization depends upon food storage and processing and upon physiological processes of nutrient absorption. Stability is then needed in expected food access – and hence stability in availability, access and utilization and in their determinants. Food security also has different dimensions as regards types of nutrient. There are also questions about the availability of cheap food. International food price spikes from 2008 have led to renewed interest in food prices and challenged the widespread observation of a steady fall in long-term real food prices. Prices have subsequently fluctuated above a base somewhat higher than pre-2008 prices. More fundamentally, however, conventional measures of 'real' food prices compare food prices with US consumer prices or the prices of manufactures', prices that are largely determined in richer economies by the demand of richer consumers and societies (with relative falls in food prices – an inevitable result of increasing incomes with economic growth). A more meaningful measure of real food prices is to compare them with incomes, which vary between rich and poor individuals and societies. Unsurprisingly, real international food prices measured in this way have not declined for poor people in the way that they have for the less poor. The studies reported above are relevant to all three pathways by which agriculture can impact on nutrition – and emphasize the relationship and overlap between them. All three pathways can involve impacts from price change and from changes in product composition, although the balance between them is likely to differ. There can also be significant complementarity, as between the development and own-production pathways, as the nutritional impacts of economic development tends to be greater in economies with greater relative importance of the agricultural sector. There is then a larger share of the workforce working in agriculture and getting a double benefit as both producers and consumers from increases in real incomes and in access to improved diets. The following steps were considered of great importance in developing a more nutrition-friendly agricultural policy:

1 Start with explicit nutrition goals
2 Clearly define the nutrition problem
3 Create and capture value for nutrition
4 Be expansive in the search for solutions, but tailor to context
5 Focus on the functioning and coordination of the whole chain in order to create sustainable solutions
6 Add value not only for nutrition (and consumers), but also for other chain actors
7 Take a broader view of adding value for producers and consumers
8 Focus on meeting, growing, and creating demand
9 Create a policy environment in which better nutrition is valued

An update on the Nutrition Related Burden of Disease was presented based on the planned *Lancet* publications to be launched early in 2013. The new series has considered the burden of undernutrition and the burden of obesity and related chronic diseases. *Lynette Neufeld* presented the concept of addressing 'malnutrition in all its forms' (underweight, wasting, stunting and overweight); micronutrient deficiencies and nutrition-related chronic diseases were also discussed and largely adopted by the group. Underweight is defined as low weight-for-age, a child may be underweight because she or he is wasted (low weight-for-height) or stunted (low height-for-age), or both. Wasting and stunting should be considered separately since they require different approaches in their treatment and control. Low birthweight is defined as being underweight at the time of birth (below 2,500 g), whereas the growth-restricted newborn is one that has low birthweight for the corresponding gestational age. Acute wasting is an important form of malnutrition, especially within the context of emergencies and child survival since it has a direct impact on resistance to infection. To attain the respective MDGs on preventing child hunger and mortality resulting from malnutrition requires successful control and prevention of malnutrition in all its forms. We clearly need new ideas leading to novel and more effective actions; research on how to best deliver these actions at the population level should also be optimized. We need to move from efficacy to true effectiveness studies under real world conditions; the search for cost-effective solutions should be the goal.

Ricardo Uauy

Black RE, Singhal A, Uauy R (eds): International Nutrition: Achieving Millennium Goals and Beyond.
Nestlé Nutr Inst Workshop Ser, vol 78, pp 59–69, (DOI: 10.1159/000354941)
Nestec Ltd., Vevey/S. Karger AG., Basel, © 2014

Interventions to Address Maternal and Childhood Undernutrition: Current Evidence

Zulfiqar A. Bhutta · Jai K. Das

Division of Women and Child Health, The Aga Khan University, Karachi, Pakistan

Abstract

The global burden of undernutrition remains high with little evidence of change in many countries. We reviewed the evidence of the potential nutritional interventions and estimated their effect on nutrition-related outcomes of women and children. Among the maternal interventions, daily iron supplementation results in a 69% reduction in incidence of anemia, 20% in incidence of low birthweight (LBW) and improves mean birthweight. MMN supplementation during pregnancy has been shown to significantly decrease the number of LBW infants by 14% and small for gestational age (SGA) by 13%. Balanced protein-energy supplementation reduces the incidence of SGA by 32% and risk of stillbirths by 38%. Antimalarials when given to pregnant women increase the mean birthweight significantly and were associated with a 43% reduction in LBW and severe antenatal anemia by 38%. Among the neonatal and child interventions, educational/counseling interventions increased exclusive breastfeeding by 43% at 4–6 weeks and 137% at 6 months. Vitamin A supplementation (VAS) reduces all-cause mortality by 24% and results in a 14% reduction in the risk of infant mortality at 6 months. Intermittent iron supplementation in children reduces the risk of anemia by 49% and iron deficiency by 76%, and significantly improves hemoglobin and ferritin concentration. Preventive zinc supplementation in populations at risk of zinc deficiency decreases morbidity from childhood diarrhea and acute lower respiratory infections, and increases linear growth and weight gain among infants and young children. Among the supportive interventions, hand washing with soap significantly reduces diarrhea morbidity by 48%, though it depends on access to water. The effect of water treatment on diarrhea morbidity also appears similarly large with a 17% reduction. Recent research has established linkages of preconception interventions with improved maternal, perinatal and neonatal health outcomes, and it has been suggested that several proven interventions recommended during pregnancy may be even more effective if implemented before conception. These proven interventions, if scaled up have the potential to reduce the global burden of undernutrition substantially.

Introduction

The State of Food Insecurity estimates that around 870 million people globally have been undernourished (in terms of dietary energy supply) in the period 2010–2012 [1]. The vast majority of these, 852 million, live in developing countries, where the prevalence of undernourishment is around 14.9% [1]. Though many countries are on track in reducing income poverty [Millennium Developmental Goal (MDG) 1a], less than a quarter of developing countries are on track to achieve the goal, of halving undernutrition (MDG 1c) by the year 2015. The global burden of undernutrition remains high with little evidence of change in many countries despite economic growth, and still millions of people are faced with starvation and malnutrition, with women and children contributing the major share. The progress has also been hampered by the global increase in food and oil prices, climate change, unprecedented draughts and increased number of countries affected by fragility, conflict and emergencies. According to the World Bank, 33 countries fall in the fragile situations category and, in addition, conflict and fragility also occur at the subnational level within some strongly performing countries. The World Bank further estimated that the food price crisis in 2008 pushed as many as 130–155 million more people globally into extreme poverty with an increase in the number of children suffering permanent cognitive and physical injury due to malnutrition by 44 million.

Malnutrition, including micronutrient deficiencies, remains one of the major public health challenges, particularly in developing countries [2]. Poor maternal nutrition contributes to at least 20% of maternal deaths, and increases the probability of other poor pregnancy outcomes including newborn deaths [2]. Low body mass index among women of reproductive age is an important risk factor for intrauterine growth restriction, low birthweight (LBW) and neonatal mortality. Other maternal indicators for poor pregnancy and neonatal outcomes include low maternal stature, anemia and other micronutrient deficiencies.

In the year 2011, almost 6.9 million children under 5 years of age died worldwide [3], and undernutrition was an underlying cause in about one third of these deaths which included stunting, severe wasting, deficiencies of vitamin A and zinc, and suboptimal breastfeeding. Globally, around 165 million children under 5 suffer from stunting, 101 million are underweight and 52 million are wast-

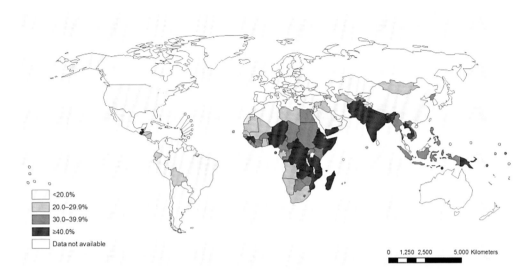

Fig. 1. Latest country prevalence estimates for stunting among children under 5 years of age. Source: http://www.who.int/nutgrowthdb/jme_unicef_who_wb.pdf.

ed, and approximately 90% of these live in just 36 countries with the highest prevalence in Southeast Asia and Sub-Saharan Africa [4] (fig. 1). Prevalence of malnourished children has decreased, and progress has been made in the past two decades, but at the current rate of progress, United Nations regional goals are unlikely to be met in all developing countries, and micronutrient deficiencies remain widespread among women and children globally.

To address this persistent burden of undernutrition in women and children and to the population at large, various strategies have been employed worldwide. Among these are nutrition education, dietary modification, food provision/supplementation, agricultural interventions including bio-fortification, micronutrient supplementation and fortification. Apart from these direct nutritional interventions, programs to tackle the underlying causes of undernutrition including prevention and management of infections (like diarrhea and malaria) have also been initiated and implemented at various levels of care. Parallel programs have also been pursued to increase coverage and aid uptake of these primary interventions including provision of financial incentives at various levels, home gardening and community-based nutrition education and mobilization programs. Although all these strategies have shown success and proved to be effective, a coherent, multifaceted and integrated action which has the global consensus is lacking, and several attempts at developing consensus is fraught with controversies and lack of coordination between various academic groups and development agencies.

Concerns for these deprived prospects have called for improved efforts to speed up and scale up the implementation of effective interventions in a systematic manner to achieve high and equitable coverage of interventions. In the following sections, we will review various interventions (table 1) and their evidence-based proven effectiveness.

Review of Interventions

Micronutrient Supplementation

The World Health Organization (WHO) estimates that in spite of recent efforts in the prevention and control of micronutrient deficiencies, over two billion people are at risk for vitamin A, iodine, and/or iron deficiency globally [5]. Other micronutrient deficiencies of public health concern include zinc, folate, and the B vitamins. In many settings, more than one micronutrient deficiency coexists, suggesting the need for simple approaches that evaluate and address multiple micronutrient (MMN) malnutrition [6]. Micronutrient supplementation is the most widely practiced intervention to prevent and manage single or MMN deficiencies. Various programs are in place to address these micronutrient deficiencies through supplementation, and evidence from evidence-based systematic reviews suggests that among pregnant women, daily iron supplementation is associated with a 69% reduction in incidence of anemia at term, 66% reduction in iron deficiency anemia at term, 20% reduction in incidence of LBW and improved birthweight [7]. Calcium supplementation during pregnancy is associated with a 52% reduction in the incidence of preeclampsia and 24% reduction in preterm birth with an increase in birthweight of 85 g, while no significant impacts were observed on perinatal mortality [8]. MMN supplementation during pregnancy significantly reduces the incidence of LBW infants by 11% and small for gestational age (SGA) by 13%. When compared with iron and folate supplementation while the impact on preterm birth, miscarriage, preeclampsia, maternal mortality, perinatal mortality, stillbirth and neonatal mortality was statistically not different [9]. Evidence of micronutrient supplementation in children indicates that vitamin A supplementation (VAS) reduces all-cause mortality and diarrhea-specific mortality by 24% and 28%, respectively [10]. VAS also reduces the incidence of diarrhea by 15% and measles morbidity by 50%; however, there was no significant effect on the incidence of respiratory disease. Iron supplementation in children results in a 49%

Table 1. Interventions to improve maternal and child undernutrition and estimates

Intervention	Estimates
Maternal interventions Iron/iron-folate supplementation	LBW (RR: 0.80, 95% CI: 0.68–0.97), birthweight (mean difference, MD: 30.81 g, 95% CI: 5.94–55.68), serum hemoglobin concentration at term (MD: 8.88 g/l, 95% CI: 6.96–10.80), anemia at term (RR: 0.31, 95% CI: 0.19–0.46), iron deficiency (RR: 0.43, 95% CI: 0.27–0.66), iron deficiency anemia (RR: 0.34, 95% CI: 0.16–0.69), side effects (RR: 2.36, 95% CI: 0.96–5.82), while nonsignificant impacts on premature delivery, neonatal death, congenital anomalies.
Maternal calcium supplementation	52% reduction in the incidence of preeclampsia (RR: 0.48, 95% CI: 0.34–0.67) with an increase in birthweight of 85 g. 24% reduction in risk of preterm birth (RR: 0.76, 95% CI: 0.60–0.97), while nonsignificant impacts on perinatal mortality, LBW and neonatal mortality.
Maternal multiple micronutrient supplementation	LBW (RR: 0.89, 95% CI: 0.83–0.94) and SGA (RR: 0.87, 95% CI: 0.81–0.95), while nonsignificant impacts on preterm birth, miscarriage, maternal mortality, perinatal mortality, stillbirths and neonatal mortality.
Maternal BEP supplementation	Reduction of 34% (RR: 0.66, 95% CI: 0.49–0.89) in the risk of SGA infants and 38% in stillbirths (RR: 0.62, 95% CI: 0.40–0.98). It also increased birthweight (MD: 73 g, 95% CI: 30–117).
Child interventions Iron supplementation	Anemia (RR: 0.51, 95% CI: 0.37–0.72), iron deficiency (RR: 0.24, 95% CI: 0.06–0.91), hemoglobin (MD: 5.20 g/l, 95% CI: 2.51–7.88), ferritin (MD: 14.17 µg/l, 95% CI: 3.53–24.81).
Vitamin A supplementation	All-cause mortality reduced by 24% (RR: 0.76, 95% CI: 0.69–0.83), diarrhea-related mortality by 28% (RR: 0.72, 95% CI: 0.57–0.91), incidence of diarrhea reduced by 15% (RR: 0.85, 95% CI: 0.82–0.87) and incidence of measles by 50% (RR: 0.50, 95% CI: 0.37–0.67), while nonsignificant impacts on measles and acute respiratory infection-related mortality.
Zinc supplementation	Height improved by 0.37 cm (SD 0.25) in children supplemented for 24 weeks, diarrhea reduced by 13%, pneumonia reduced by 19%, while nonsignificant impacts on mortality.
Breastfeeding	EBF increase by 43% at 4–6 weeks with 89 and 20% significant increases in developing and developed countries, respectively. EBF also improves at 6 months by 137%, with six times increase in developing countries.
Complementary/ supplementary feeding	Statistically significant difference of effect for length during the intervention in children.

Table 1. Continued

Intervention	Estimates
Disease prevention and management	
WASH interventions	Diarrhea risk reductions of 48% (RR: 0.52, 95% CI: 0.34–0.65) with hand washing with soap, 17% with improved water quality and 36% with excreta disposal.
Deworming	Prophylactic single- and multiple-dose deworming had a nonsignificant effect on hemoglobin and weight gain. Treating children with proven infection showed that single dose of deworming drugs increases weight (MD: 0.58 kg, 95% CI: 0.40–0.76) and hemoglobin (MD: 0.37 g/dl, 95% CI: 0.1–0.64).
Malaria prevention and treatment	Antimalarials to prevent malaria in pregnant women reduced antenatal parasitemia (RR: 0.53, 95% CI: 0.33–0.86), increased birthweight (MD: 126.7 g, 95% CI: 88.64–164.75), reduced LBW and severe antenatal anemia by 43 and 38%, respectively. Insecticide-treated mosquito nets in pregnancy reduced LBW by 23% (RR: 0.77, 95% CI: 0.61–0.98) and reduced fetal loss (1st to 4th pregnancy), by 33% (RR: 0.67, 95% CI: 0.47–0.97), while there was a nonsignificant impacts on anemia and clinical malaria.

lower risk of anemia and a 74% lower risk of iron deficiency with higher serum hemoglobin and ferritin concentration, while nonsignificant impacts were observed for height-for-age and weight-for-age [11]. Zinc supplementation at a dose of 10 mg zinc/day for 24 weeks could lead to a net gain in height of 0.37 cm (±0.25) [12] and reduce the incidence of diarrhea by 13% and pneumonia morbidity by 19%, while has nonsignificant effects on mortality [13]. MMN supplementation with 3 or more micronutrients in children showed small effect sizes for length/height and weight, with limited evidence for an impact on outcomes such as morbidity and cognitive function [14].

Micronutrient Fortification and Agricultural Interventions

Food fortification is a strategy that has been used safely and effectively to prevent vitamin and mineral deficiencies. It has the advantage of reaching a wider at-risk population through existing food delivery systems, without requiring major changes in existing consumption patterns and also is cost-effective. Many programs have been initiated and are in place, but few have been formally evaluated to assess its actual impact. A review of MMN fortification in children showed an increase in hemoglobin levels and a 57% reduced risk of anemia. Fortification is also associated with increased vitamin A serum levels. A review on mass salt fortification with vitamin A and iodine concluded that the fortified and iodized salt can improve the iodine status [15]. Zinc and vitamin D fortification has been effective, as evaluated by various programs. The evidence from developing countries however is scarce, and these programs also need to assess the direct impact of fortification on morbidity and mortality.

Bio-fortification is a relatively new strategy to improve iron, zinc, and vitamin A status in low-income populations. It is the use of conventional breeding techniques and biotechnology to improve the micronutrient quality of staple crops. A review on bio-fortification concluded that it has the potential to contribute to increased micronutrient intakes and improve micronutrient status; however, this domain requires further research [16].

Agricultural interventions including home and school gardening also have potential. A review on agricultural interventions to improve nutritional status of children concluded that home gardening interventions had a positive effect on the production of the agricultural goods and consumption of food rich in protein and micronutrients. Some evidence of a positive effect on absorption of vitamin A was also observed. However, the impacts on iron absorption and anthropometric indices remained inconclusive [17].

Improving Feeding and Energy Intake

Besides the micronutrient supplementation, macronutrient interventions have also been proposed and evaluated in accordance with the maternal needs during pregnancy, which includes dietary advice, balanced protein-energy (BEP) supplementation and high protein, isocaloric protein supplementation. A review [18] shows that providing pregnant females with BEP supplementation results in a significant reduction of 34% in the risk of giving birth to an SGA infant and 38% reduction in stillbirth, and results in an increased birthweight. These effects were more pronounced in malnourished women when compared to adequately nourished women.

In children, improved feeding in early infancy and the initial years of life holds an utmost importance, and breastfeeding and complementary feeding are strategies which ensure optimum nutrition during this vital phase of growth and development. Breastmilk provides numerous immunologic, psychologic, social, economic and environmental benefits; it is a natural first food and ideal nutrition for the newborn [19]. Breastfeeding is therefore recommended as the optimal strategy for feeding newborns and young infants. Strategies to improve the uptake of breastfeeding are essential, and evidence suggests that breastfeeding education and promotion interventions are effective in improving breastfeeding rates and are associated with improved exclusive breastfeeding rates (EBF) of 43% at 4–6 weeks, with 89 and 20% significant increases in developing and developed countries, respectively. EBF also improved at 6 months by 137%, with six times increase in developing countries compared to a 1.3-fold increase in developed countries [20].

Complementary feeding for infants refers to the timely introduction of safe and nutritional foods in addition to breastfeeding, typically provided to children from 6 to 24 months of age [21]. Multiple complementary nutrition interventions targeted to improve nutritional status of children have been reviewed. These include complementary and supplementary feeding programs with or without nutrition education. Dewey and Adu-Afarwuah [22] reviewed the effectiveness and efficacy of complementary feeding interventions in children aged 6–24 months in developing countries and indicated that provision of complementary food can have a significant impact on growth under well-controlled situations. Complementary food combined with maternal education improved weight and linear growth. A recent review [23] looking at the impact of supplementary feeding that covered energy-protein supplementation found a statistically significant difference of effect for length during the intervention in children aged less than 12 years of age.

Disease Prevention and Management

Recurrent illnesses contribute to undernutrition burden, and strategies devised at the prevention and treatment of recurrent infections can contribute to addressing the existing undernutrition. These include the Water, Sanitation and Hygiene (WASH) interventions, interventions for prevention and treatment of diarrhea and malaria.

A review drawing upon three systematic reviews focused on the effect of hand washing with soap on diarrhea, of water quality improvement and of excreta disposal. It concluded that hand washing with soap significantly reduces diarrhea morbidity by 48%. The effect of improved water quality on diarrhea morbidity also appears similarly large with a 17% reduction, while there is very little rigorous evidence for the health benefit of sanitation [24].

WHO recommends that all schoolchildren should be treated at regular intervals with deworming drugs in helminthic-prevalent areas. A recent review

[25] shows that treating children after screening for worms with a single dose of deworming drugs may increase weight and hemoglobin. Administration of a single dose of antihelminthics in the second trimester of pregnancy failed to show a statistically significant impact on maternal anemia or LBW, preterm births and perinatal mortality. Effective interventions to prevent malaria morbidity and mortality include insecticide-treated mosquito nets, indoor-residual spraying and intermittent preventive therapy. A review [26] concludes that antimalarials when given to prevent malaria in pregnant women increased mean birthweight and reduced the incidence of LBW by 43% and severe antenatal anemia by 38% [26]. Therapeutic zinc supplementation for the management of diarrhea reduces all-cause mortality by 46% and diarrhea-related hospitalization by 23% [27].

Conclusion

We have the evidence for multiple interventions which work at various levels of care and, if implemented at scale, have the potential to reduce undernutrition burden globally. The long-term sustainability of such programs, however, is hindered in developing countries because of government policies, human resource constraints, bad communication networks including roads and the fragile health system infrastructure and participant compliance. Hence, the universal coverage with the full package of proven interventions could be the way forward in achieving the MDGs. Another important factor to consider is the cost-effectiveness of the proposed package. In the Copenhagen consensus statement 2012 [28], it was concluded that for about USD 100 per child, a bundle of interventions including micronutrient provision, complementary foods, treatments for worms and diarrheal diseases, and behavior change programs, could reduce chronic undernutrition by 36% in developing countries. Even in very poor countries, each dollar spent reducing chronic undernutrition has at least a USD 30 payoff.

All that is required is a global consensus on the package of interventions to be implemented and an agreed upon mode of delivery which ensures effective uptake and access to populations who need it most.

Disclosure Statement

No financial disclosures.

References

1 Food and Agriculture Organization of the United Nations: The state of food insecurity in the world. Economic growth is necessary but not sufficient to accelerate reduction of hunger and malnutrition. Rome, Food and Agriculture Organization of the United Nations, 2012.

2 Black RE, Allen LH, Bhutta ZA, et al: Maternal and child undernutrition: global and regional exposures and health consequences. Lancet 2008;371:243–260.

3 UNICEF, WHO, The World Bank, UN: Levels and trends in child mortality: 2012 report. New York, United Nations Children's Fund, 2012.

4 UNICEF, WHO, The World Bank: Joint child malnutrition estimates – levels and trends. New York, World Health Organization, 2012.

5 World Health Organization: World health report, 2000. Geneva, World Health Organization, 2000.

6 Ramakrishnan U: Prevalence of micronutrient malnutrition worldwide. Nutr Rev 2002; 5:S46–S52.

7 Imdad A, Bhutta ZA: Routine iron/folate supplementation during pregnancy: effect on maternal anaemia and birth outcomes. Paediatr Perinat Epidemiol 2012;26(suppl 1):168–177.

8 Imdad A, Bhutta ZA: Effects of calcium supplementation during pregnancy on maternal, fetal and birth outcomes. Paediatr Perinat Epidemiol 2012;26(suppl 1):138–152.

9 Haider BA, Bhutta ZA: Multiple micronutrient supplementation for women during pregnancy. Cochrane Database Syst Rev 2012;CD004905.

10 Imdad A, Herzer K, Mayo-Wilson E, Yakoob MY, Bhutta ZA: Vitamin A supplementation for preventing morbidity and mortality in children from 6 months to 5 years of age. Cochrane Database Syst Rev 2010;CD008524.

11 De-Regil LM, Jefferds ME, Sylvetsky AC, Dowswell T: Intermittent iron supplementation for improving nutrition and development in children under 12 years of age. Cochrane Database Syst Rev 2011;CD009085.

12 Imdad A, Bhutta Z: Effect of preventive zinc supplementation on linear growth in children under 5 years of age in developing countries: a meta-analysis of studies for input to the lives saved tool. BMC Public Health 2011; 11(suppl 3):S22.

13 Yakoob MY, Theodoratou E, Jabeen A, et al: Preventive zinc supplementation in developing countries: impact on mortality and morbidity due to diarrhea, pneumonia and malaria. BMC Public Health 2011;11(suppl 3):S23.

14 Christian P, Tielsch JM: Evidence for multiple micronutrient effects based on randomized controlled trials and meta-analyses in developing countries. J Nutr 2011;142:173S–177S.

15 Jiang T, Xue Q: Fortified salt for preventing iodine deficiency disorders: a systematic review. Chin J Evid Based Med 2010;10:857–861.

16 Hotz C, McClafferty B: From harvest to health: challenges for developing biofortified staple foods and determining their impact on micronutrient status. Food Nutr Bull 2007; 28(suppl 2):S271–S279.

17 Masset E, Haddad L, Cornelius A, Isaza-Castro J: Effectiveness of agricultural interventions that aim to improve nutritional status of children: systematic review. BMJ 2012; 344:d8222.

18 Imdad A, Bhutta ZA: Effect of balanced protein energy supplementation during pregnancy on birth outcomes. BMC Public Health 2011;11(suppl 3):S17.

19 Dewey KG, Heinig MJ, Nommsen LA, et al: Growth of breast-fed and formula-fed infants from 0 to 18 months: the DARLING study. Pediatrics 1992;89:1035–1041.

20 Imdad A, Yakoob MY, Bhutta ZA: Effect of breastfeeding promotion interventions on breastfeeding rates, with special focus on developing countries. BMC Public Health 2011; 11(suppl 3):S24.

21 World Health Organization: Report of informal meeting to review and develop indicators for complementary feeding. Washington, World Health Organization, 2002.

22 Dewey KG, Adu-Afarwuah S: Systematic review of the efficacy and effectiveness of complementary feeding interventions in developing countries. Matern Child Nutr 2008; 4(suppl 1):24–85.

23 Sguassero Y, de Onis M, Bonotti AM, Carroli G: Community-based supplementary feeding for promoting the growth of children under five years of age in low and middle income countries. Cochrane Database Syst Rev 2012;CD005039.

24 Cairncross S, Hunt C, Boisson S, et al: Water, sanitation and hygiene for the prevention of diarrhoea. Int J Epidemiol 2010;39(suppl 1): i193–i205.

25 Taylor-Robinson D, Jones A, Garner P: Deworming drugs for treating soil-transmitted intestinal worms in children: effects on growth and school performance. Cochrane Database Syst Rev 2012;CD000371.

26 Garner P, Gülmezoglu AM: Drugs for preventing malaria in pregnant women. Cochrane Database Syst Rev 2009;CD000169.

27 Walker CLF, Black RE: Zinc for the treatment of diarrhoea: effect on diarrhoea morbidity, mortality and incidence of future episodes. Int J Epidemiol 2010;39(suppl 1):i63–i69.

28 Copenhagen Consensus Center: Copenhagen Consensus 2012: Solving the World's Challenges.

Evidence on Interventions and Field Experiences

Black RE, Singhal A, Uauy R (eds): International Nutrition: Achieving Millennium Goals and Beyond.
Nestlé Nutr Inst Workshop Ser, vol 78, pp 71–80, (DOI: 10.1159/000354942)
Nestec Ltd., Vevey/S. Karger AG., Basel, © 2014

Maternal Nutrition Interventions to Improve Maternal, Newborn, and Child Health Outcomes

Usha Ramakrishnan · Beth Imhoff-Kunsch · Reynaldo Martorell

Hubert Department of Global Health, Rollins School of Public Health, and Nutrition & Health
Sciences Program, Graduate Division of Biological & Biomedical Sciences, Emory University,
Atlanta, GA, USA

Abstract

Maternal undernutrition affects a large proportion of women in many developing countries, but has received little attention as an important determinant of poor maternal, newborn, and child health (MNCH) outcomes such as intrauterine growth restriction, preterm birth (PTB), and maternal and infant morbidity and mortality. We recently evaluated the scientific evidence on the effects of maternal nutrition interventions on MNCH outcomes as part of a project funded by the Gates Foundation to identify critical knowledge gaps and priority research needs. A standardized tool was used for study data abstraction, and the effect of nutrition interventions during pregnancy or of factors such as interpregnancy interval on MNCH outcomes was assessed by meta-analysis, when possible. Several nutrient interventions provided during pregnancy have beneficial effects on MNCH outcomes, but are not widely adopted. For example, prenatal calcium supplementation decreases the risk of PTB and increases birthweight; prenatal zinc, omega-3 fatty acids and multiple micronutrient supplements reduce the risk of PTB (<37 weeks), early PTB (<34 weeks) and low birthweight (LBW), respectively. Among currently implemented interventions, balanced protein-energy and iron-folic acid supplementation during pregnancy significantly reduce the risk of LBW by 20–30% in controlled settings, but variable programmatic experiences have led to questionable effectiveness. Early age at pregnancy and short interpregnancy intervals were also associated with increased risk of PTB, LBW and neonatal death, but major gaps remain on the role of women's nutrition before and during early pregnancy and nutrition education and counseling. These findings emphasize the need to examine the benefits of improving maternal nutrition before and during pregnancy both in research and program delivery.

© 2014 Nestec Ltd., Vevey/S. Karger AG, Basel

Introduction

Maternal, newborn, and child health (MNCH) outcomes such as anemia, intra-uterine growth restriction (IUGR), low birthweight (LBW), and preterm birth (PTB) remain major public health problems that are associated with significant costs to health care and human capital formation [1]. Preeclampsia, one of the leading causes of maternal morbidity and mortality worldwide, can lead to poor health outcomes for both the mother (e.g. damage to vital organs) and her child (e.g. IUGR, PTB) [2]. Although considerable strides and investments have been made in improving child health and survival, the importance of maternal and child nutrition especially during the first 1,000 days that begin in utero through the first year of life has received attention only recently [3, 4]. Maternal nutrition before and during pregnancy is especially important for healthy pregnancy outcomes in many lower and middle-income countries (LMIC), where women enter pregnancy undernourished and their nutritional status worsens throughout pregnancy due to the increased demand for nutrients [5]. For example, anemia is widespread among women of reproductive age in many LMIC. Anemia during pregnancy, especially severe anemia which is often due to iron deficiency, has been linked to poor health outcomes such as LBW, PTB, maternal morbidities, and maternal and child mortality [6]. Several public health programs have strived to reduce the prevalence of anemia, especially in high-risk areas, but these efforts have not translated to improved outcomes often due to poor program implementation and/or inadequate support for maternal health. Inadequate food intake in terms quantity and quality combined with high prevalences of underweight and/or short stature has also been associated with poor MNCH outcomes in some settings [7, 8].

This review examines the state of current knowledge on the impact of nutrition-related interventions for women before and during pregnancy on MNCH outcomes including IUGR, LBW, PTB, newborn and child growth, morbidity and mortality, and maternal morbidity and mortality with recommendations for programs and research.

Methods

We based the present review on a recently published collection of meta-analyses examining the effect of maternal nutrition on a broad range of MNCH outcomes, with a particular focus on nutrition interventions during pregnancy [9]. The meta-analyses describe interventions during pregnancy, pre-pregnancy interventions, and nutrition throughout the life cycle. Authors conducted the meta-analyses and comprehensive literature reviews using evidence from randomized controlled trials (RCTs) and/or observational studies. Although the meta-analyses primarily focused on nutrition interventions during preg-

Table 1. Number of prenatal nutrition intervention trials included in each meta-analysis, by intervention and outcome

	Calcium	Iodine	Iron or IFA	Zinc	Vit A	Vit D	Vit B$_6$	Vit B$_{12}$	Vit C (+E)	n-3 PUFA	MMN	Balanced protein-energy
PTB	11	–	12	16	7	2	–	–	9	9	9	6
LBW	6	–	11	11	5	3	–	–	5	8	15	5
Birthweight	13	2	13	20	7	5	3	–	8	9	14	16
Neonatal or infant mortality	2	2	4	–	5	–	–	–	9	6	9	3
Anemia	–	–	18	–	8	–	–	–	–	–	7	–
PIH or preeclampsia	15	–	2	–	–	–	2	–	9	4	–	3
Maternal mortality	–	–	–	–	3	–	–	–	–	–	2	–

Dashes indicate not reported or very low-quality/insufficient data. PIH = Pregnancy-induced hypertension.

nancy, the topics of antihelminthics in pregnancy, nutrition education and counseling, household food production, short interpregnancy interval, early age at first childbirth, nutrition before and during pregnancy, and intergenerational influences on child growth and undernutrition were included because of their potential impact on maternal and child health outcomes [10–16]. We reviewed meta-analyses of the following specific supplementation trials during pregnancy: iron or iron + folic acid (IFA), vitamin A, select B vitamins, vitamin D, n-3 long-chain polyunsaturated fatty acids (n-3 PUFA), iodine, zinc, calcium, multiple micronutrient (MMN), balanced protein-energy, and antihelminthics [10, 17–27]. For all reviews, authors abstracted study data using a standardized Excel-based tool that captured information on 49 potential variables, for example sample size, study design, study context, and estimated effect [9]. Authors graded the quality of evidence for each intervention, where data were available, using the Child Health Epidemiology Reference Group's (CHERG) adaptation of the GRADE methodology as a guide [28, 29].

Results

The results of findings for nutrition interventions during pregnancy and nutrition-sensitive interventions before and during pregnancy are described in the following sections.

Nutrition Interventions during Pregnancy

A summary of the number of individual trials included in the meta-analyses of nutrition interventions during pregnancy is given by type of intervention and outcome in table 1. The number of trials ranged from 0 to 20 and varied by type

Table 2. Effect of select nutrition interventions during pregnancy on newborn outcomes[1]

	Birthweight, g		LBW		PTB	
	trials (total)	mean difference (95% CI)	trials (total)	pooled RR (95% CI)	trials (total)	pooled RR (95% CI)
Calcium	13 (8,574)	86 (38–134)	6 (14,479)	0.85 (0.72–1.01)	11 (15,275)	0.76 (0.60–0.97)
Iron or IFA	13 (NR)	42 (9–75)	12 (9,397)	0.80 (0.71–0.90)	12 (NR)	0.94 (0.84–1.06)
Zinc	20 (8,138)	13 (–9 to 35)	11 (5,614)	1.06 (0.91–1.23)	16 (7,818)	0.86 (0.75–0.99)
n-3 PUFA	9 (6,020)	42 (15–70)	8 (6,511)	0.92 (0.83–1.02)	5 (4,343)[2]	0.74 (0.58–0.94)[2]
MMN	15 (NR)	53 (43–62)	16 (4,040)	0.86 (0.81–0.91)	9 (9,876)	0.99 (0.96–1.03)
Balanced protein-energy	16 (6,474)	74 (30–117)	5 (4,196)	0.68 (0.51–0.92)	6 (3,579)	0.96 (0.80–1.15)

NR = Not reported.
[1] Overall moderate- to high-quality evidence.
[2] Early PTB.

of intervention and outcome measured. Several trials were identified for interventions such as zinc, calcium, IFA, MMN and balanced protein-energy. In contrast, there have been no trials of vitamin B_{12} supplementation during pregnancy, and very few trials of prenatal vitamin B_6, vitamin D, and iodine supplementation. The majority of included trials reported more information on newborn outcomes such as LBW, birthweight, and PTB than on maternal outcomes. There were also differences in the nature of the intervention received by the treatment and control groups, especially for the trials that evaluated multinutrient interventions. The MMN trials used IFA as the control group, and the authors defined MMN as 5 or more micronutrients. A mix of interventions and controls were used in the balanced protein-energy trials (e.g. in some trials both groups received micronutrients, in other trials only the intervention group received micronutrients), and zinc was often provided in addition to other micronutrients (e.g. zinc + MMN vs. MMN alone). Vitamins C and E were given concurrently in the included vitamin C trials.

Table 2 lists key results on the effect of maternal nutrition interventions on newborn outcomes. Supplementation with calcium, balanced protein-energy, MMN, IFA, or n-3 PUFA resulted in a significant ($p < 0.05$) mean increase in birthweight, compared to controls (42–86 g higher). Babies born to mothers supplemented with IFA, MMN, or balanced protein-energy had a lower risk of being born LBW than controls. Calcium and zinc supplementation significantly decreased the risk of PTB (<37 weeks), while n-3 PUFA supplementation decreased the risk of early PTB (<34 weeks). Prenatal supplementation with vitamin A decreased the risk of LBW in a subpopulation of HIV+ women (RR: 0.79,

Ramakrishnan · Imhoff-Kunsch · Martorell

Table 3. Effect of nutrition interventions during pregnancy on maternal health outcomes

	Anemia		PIH		Preeclampsia	
	trials (total)	pooled RR (95% CI)	trials (total)	pooled RR (95% CI)	trials (total)	pooled RR (95% CI)
Calcium	–	–	12 (NR)	0.65 (0.53–0.81)	15 (16,490)	0.48 (0.34–0.67)
Iron or IFA	18 (8,665)	0.31 (0.22–0.44)	–	–	2 (NR)	2.58 (0.81–8.22)
Vitamin A	8 (1,587)	0.81 (0.69–0.94)	–	–	–	–
Vitamin C + E	–	–	5 (17,353)	1.10 (1.02–1.19)	9 (19,798)	1.00 (0.91–1.10)
n-3 PUFA	–	–	5 (1,831)	1.09 (0.90–1.33)	4 (1,683)	0.86 (0.59–1.27)
MMN[1]	7 (1,299)	1.03 (0.94–1.12)	–	–	–	–

Dashes indicate not reported or very low-quality/insufficient data.
[1] Control group was IFA.

95% CI: 0.64–0.99; data from 3 RCTs), but no significant effect was found in the total population [18]. High-quality evidence demonstrates that prenatal iodine supplementation decreased the risk of cretinism (RR: 0.27, 95% CI: 0.12–0.60; data from 5 RCTs) and improved developmental scores (data from 4 RCTs) in children born to mothers at risk of iodine deficiency [22]. Evidence also suggests that prenatal iodine supplementation decreased the rate of infant mortality (data from 2 RCTs, total n = 37,400). Supplementation with vitamin B_6 resulted in higher mean birthweight; however, small sample size and poor study quality render this estimate unreliable [19].

Table 3 shows key, though limited, results of the effect of nutrition interventions on maternal outcomes. Of note, calcium supplementation decreased the risk of preeclampsia, pregnancy-induced hypertension, and maternal mortality/severe morbidity [24]. Iron or IFA and vitamin A significantly decreased the risk of maternal anemia [17, 18], but MMN interventions did not further reduce the risk of anemia compared to IFA [27]. We did not find any evidence of benefit for maternal mortality that was based on fewer trials (n = 5) that examined the effects of vitamin A (RR: 0.86, 95% CI: 0.6–1.24; 3 trials) and MMN interventions (RR: 0.96, 95% CI: 0.64–1.45; 2 trials) [18, 25].

Nutrition-Related Factors before and during Pregnancy

These topics include nutrition education and counseling during pregnancy, household food production strategies, increasing interpregnancy interval, early age at first childbirth and women's nutritional status before and during early pregnancy. Data from well-controlled trials were limited for many of these out-

Table 4. Effect of nutrition-related interventions during pregnancy on MNCH outcomes[1]

	Anemia		PTB		LBW		Birthweight, g	
	trials or studies (total)	pooled RR or aOR (95% CI)	trials or studies (total)	pooled RR or aOR (95% CI)	trials or studies (total)	pooled RR or aOR (95% CI)	trials or studies (total)	mean difference (95% CI)
Antihelminthics	3 (2,035)	0.93 (0.79–1.10)	–	–	2 (1,942)	0.21 (0.05–0.83)[2]	2 (1,942)	3.2 (–40.4 to 46.7)
Nutrition education and counseling	11 (2,588)	0.70 (0.58–0.84)	10 (3,384)	0.81 (0.66–0.99)	12 (4,311)	0.86 (0.70–1.04)	13 (1,724)	105.2 (17.7–192.7)
Short interpregnancy interval	–	–	6 (126,863)	1.41 (1.20–1.65)[3]	5 (98,508)	1.44 (1.30–1.61)[3]	–	–
Early age at first childbirth	8 (36,197)	1.36 (1.24–1.49)	23 (310,702)	1.68 (1.34–2.11)	9 (263,721)	1.39 (1.23–1.58)[1]	–	–

Dashes indicate not reported or very low-quality/insufficient data.
[1] Estimates presented in this table are of moderate to low quality due to the heterogeneity of study design and analytical methods.
[2] Very LBW.
[3] Interpregnancy interval <6 months.

comes. In cases where it was not possible to conduct an RCT due to the nature of the topic, authors used data from high-quality observational studies to conduct meta-analyses. Authors carried out a meta-analysis of antihelminthics during pregnancy; however, few RCTs have been conducted. The topics of preconception nutrition intergenerational influences on child growth and nutrition were presented as reviews.

Table 4 shows results from the meta-analyses of factors that may influence MNCH outcomes. Antihelminthics in pregnancy reduced the risk of very LBW; however, the meta-analysis included only 2 trials (1,936 women). Nutrition education and counseling resulted in improvements in various MNCH outcomes (anemia, PTB and birthweight). Early age at first childbirth and short interpregnancy interval significantly increased the odds of PTB and LBW. Early age at first childbirth also resulted in increased odds of stillbirth (aOR: 1.35, 95% CI: 1.07–1.71) and early neonatal death (aOR: 1.29, 95% CI: 1.02–1.64) [8]. Four studies examining household food production strategies as a means to improve nutritional status focused mainly on child malnutrition as an outcome and found no effect on stunting, underweight, or wasting [11]. The analyses of nutrition education and counseling, household food production strategies, short interpregnancy interval, and early age at first childbirth included studies that varied in quality and were quite methodologically heterogeneous.

The review on the role of women's nutrition before and during pregnancy found high-quality evidence supporting the importance of folate during the periconceptional period in reducing the risk of neural tube defects and suggestive of reductions for other birth defects such as congenital anomalies. The evidence from observational studies that examined women's nutritional status based on anthropometry and/or micronutrient status suggests possible benefits for outcomes such as PTB and LBW, but the studies were of poor quality, and there were no well-designed trials [15]. In contrast, evidence from long-term follow-up studies strongly supports that investing in strategies to improve child nutrition during the first few years of life results in improved maternal nutritional status later on, which may be linked to improved birth outcomes for the next generation [16].

Discussion and Conclusions

We reviewed results from a recent collection of meta-analyses examining the role of maternal, and especially prenatal, nutrition interventions on MNCH outcomes [9]. Meta-analyses of intervention trials showed that prenatal supplementation with calcium, IFA, n-3 PUFA, MMN, or balanced protein-energy resulted in higher mean birthweight, compared to controls. Prenatal supplementation with calcium, zinc, and n-3 PUFA also lowered the risk of PTB, and iron, MMN, and balanced protein-energy supplementation resulted in a lower risk of LBW. There was strong evidence that prenatal calcium supplementation decreased the risk of preeclampsia, and that IFA supplementation decreased the risk of anemia. Nutrition education and counseling during pregnancy is a promising strategy to improve maternal nutrition, although more well-designed studies are needed to estimate the cost-effectiveness and barriers to implementation of this public health strategy. Analysis of observational study data for the topics of nutrition education and counseling, household food production strategies, interpregnancy interval, and early age at first childbirth was more often than not limited by heterogeneity of study design and analytical methodology.

This review helped identify existing interventions that work and need to be strengthened with improved program implementation, new interventions that are efficacious but not widely implemented, and finally important gaps that need to be addressed in future research to generate findings that will help guide policy and programs. The provision of iodine using iodized salt and/or supplements is the most successful intervention to date, but constant monitoring is still needed. Balanced protein-energy and IFA supplementation during pregnancy are also important existing interventions that can significantly improve MNCH outcomes but face programmatic challenges. Solutions to address barriers related to program delivery, costs and scaling up are needed to improve effectiveness in settings where food insecurity and poor access to care are common. Innovative approaches that evaluate targeting, nutrition education and cash transfer programs should be pursued.

The interventions that have promise for future implementation are the provision of MMN supplements, calcium and omega-3 fatty acids during pregnancy, but these interventions need more testing in programmatic settings in LMIC. MMN interventions are safe and efficacious, but earlier concerns about possible adverse effects on neonatal mortality and issues related to the dose and composition of these supplements remain hurdles to implementation. Calcium supplementation shows evident benefit in trials, and implementation research is urgently needed given that the problem of preeclampsia is serious and widespread in both developing and developed countries. In the case of omega-3 fatty acids, most of the research has been done in developed countries rather than LMIC, where the impact of supplementation may be greater. Hence, more n-3 PUFA supplementation trials are needed in LMIC. Cost-effective ways of delivering the above interventions are also needed.

Finally, this review also identified major research gaps as outlined below:
- Dearth of evidence on several maternal outcomes
- Few antihelminthics trials – this is unfortunate because this problem is widespread in many regions of the world and the intervention is amenable to an RCT design
- More rigorous, controlled, balanced protein-energy trials also including micronutrients, fatty acids, etc. (i.e. fortified foods) and/or nutrition counseling should be considered along with additional outcomes
- Well-designed observational studies that examine the relationships between pre-pregnancy body size and composition and MNCH outcomes are needed
- The relationships between nutrition and infection during early pregnancy for predicting subsequent outcomes is unclear
- Efficacy of balanced protein-energy and/or micronutrient interventions (IFA, MMN) before and during early pregnancy on MNCH outcomes

Future research that evaluates the benefits of improving women's nutrition before and during pregnancy is critical to having better informed strategies that will help reduce the burden of outcomes such LBW, PTB and maternal and neonatal mortality, especially in settings where underlying issues such as poverty, food insecurity and gender discrimination remain.

Disclosure Statement

The authors declare that no financial or other conflict of interest exists in relation to the content of the chapter.

References

1 Victora CG, Adair L, Fall C, et al: Maternal and child undernutrition: consequences for adult health and human capital. Lancet 2008; 371:340–357.

2 Villar J, Purwar M, Merialdi M, et al: World Health Organisation multicentre randomised trial of supplementation with vitamins C and E among pregnant women at high risk for pre-eclampsia in populations of low nutritional status from developing countries. Br J Obstet Gynaecol 2009;116:780–788.

3 Kind KL, Moore VM, Davies MJ: Diet around conception and during pregnancy – effects on fetal and neonatal outcomes. Reprod Biomed Online 2006;12:532–541.

4 Vobecky JS: Nutritional aspects of preconceptional period as related to pregnancy and early infancy. Prog Food Nutr Sci 1986;10: 205–236.

5 Bhutta ZA, Haider BA: Maternal micronutrient deficiencies in developing countries. Lancet 2008;371:186–187.

6 Ramakrishnan U, Imhoff-Kunsch B: Anemia and iron deficiency in developing countries; in Lammi Keefe CJ, Couch SC, Philipson EH (eds): Handbook of Nutrition and Pregnancy, Nutrition and Health. Totowa, Humana Press, 2008, pp 337–354.

7 Ronnenberg AG, Wang X, Xing H, et al: Low preconception body mass index is associated with birth outcome in a prospective cohort of Chinese women. J Nutr 2003;133:3449–3455.

8 Subramaniam SV, Ackerson LK, Smith GD, John NA: Association of maternal height with child mortality, anthropometric failure, and anemia in India. JAMA 2009;301:1691–1701.

9 Imhoff-Kunsch B, Martorell R: Nutrition interventions during pregnancy and maternal, newborn and child health outcomes. Paediatr Perinat Epidemiol 2012;26(suppl 1):1–3.

10 Imhoff-Kunsch B, Briggs V: Antihelminthics in pregnancy and maternal, newborn and child health. Paediatr Perinat Epidemiol 2012;26(suppl 1):223–238.

11 Girard AW, Olude O: Nutrition education and counselling provided during pregnancy: effects on maternal, neonatal and child health outcomes. Paediatr Perinat Epidemiol 2012; 26(suppl 1):191–204.

12 Girard AW, Self JL, McAuliffe C, et al: The effects of household food production strategies on the health and nutrition outcomes of women and young children: a systematic review. Paediatr Perinat Epidemiol 2012; 26(suppl 1):205–222.

13 Wendt A, Gibbs CM, Peters S, et al: Impact of increasing inter-pregnancy interval on maternal and infant health. Paediatr Perinat Epidemiol 2012;26(suppl 1):239–258.

14 Gibbs CM, Wendt A, Peters S, et al: The impact of early age at first childbirth on maternal and infant health. Paediatr Perinat Epidemiol 2012;26(suppl 1):259–284.

15 Ramakrishnan U, Grant F, Goldenberg T, et al: Effect of women's nutrition before and during early pregnancy on maternal and infant outcomes: a systematic review. Paediatr Perinat Epidemiol 2012;26(suppl 1):285–301.

16 Martorell R, Zongrone A: Intergenerational influences on child growth and undernutrition. Paediatr Perinat Epidemiol 2012; 26(suppl 1):302–314.

17 Imdad A, Bhutta ZA: Routine iron/folate supplementation during pregnancy: effect on maternal anaemia and birth outcomes. Paediatr Perinat Epidemiol 2012;26(suppl 1):168–177.

18 Thorne-Lyman AL, Fawzi WW: Vitamin A and carotenoids during pregnancy and maternal, neonatal and infant health outcomes: a systematic review and meta-analysis. Paediatr Perinat Epidemiol 2012;26(suppl 1):36–54.

19 Dror DK, Allen LH: Interventions with vitamins B6, B12 and C in pregnancy. Paediatr Perinat Epidemiol 2012;26(suppl 1):55–74.

20 Thorne-Lyman A, Fawzi WW: Vitamin D during pregnancy and maternal, neonatal and infant health outcomes: a systematic review and meta-analysis. Paediatr Perinat Epidemiol 2012;26(suppl 1):75–90.

21 Imhoff-Kunsch B, Briggs V, Goldenberg T: Effect of n-3 long-chain polyunsaturated fatty acid intake during pregnancy on maternal, infant, and child health outcomes: a systematic review. Paediatr Perinat Epidemiol 2012; 26(suppl 1):91–107.

22 Zimmermann MB: The effects of iodine deficiency in pregnancy and infancy. Paediatr Perinat Epidemiol 2012;26(suppl 1):108–117.

23 Chaffee BW, King JC: Effect of zinc supplementation on pregnancy and infant outcomes: a systematic review. Paediatr Perinat Epidemiol 2012;26(suppl 1):118–137.

24 Imdad A, Bhutta ZA: Effects of calcium supplementation during pregnancy on maternal, fetal and birth outcomes. Paediatr Perinat Epidemiol 2012;26(suppl 1):138–152.

25 Ramakrishnan U, Grant FK, Goldenberg T, et al: Effect of multiple micronutrient supplementation on pregnancy and infant outcomes: a systematic review. Paediatr Perinat Epidemiol 2012;26(suppl 1):153–167.

26 Imdad A, Bhutta ZA: Maternal nutrition and birth outcomes: effect of balanced protein-energy supplementation. Paediatr Perinat Epidemiol 2012;26(suppl 1):178–190.

27 Bhutta ZA, Imdad SA, Ramakrishnan U, Martorell R: Is it time to replace iron folate supplements in pregnancy with multiple micronutrients? Paediatr Perinat Epidemiol 2012;26(suppl 1):27–35.

28 Atkins D, Best D, Briss PA, et al: Grading quality of evidence and strength of recommendations. BMJ 2004;328:1490–1494.

29 Walker N, Fischer-Walker C, Bryce J, et al: Standards for CHERG reviews of intervention effects on child survival. Int J Epidemiol 2010;39:2.

Black RE, Singhal A, Uauy R (eds): International Nutrition: Achieving Millennium Goals and Beyond.
Nestlé Nutr Inst Workshop Ser, vol 78, pp 81–91, (DOI: 10.1159/000354943)
Nestec Ltd., Vevey/S. Karger AG., Basel, © 2014

Fetal Growth Restriction and Preterm as Determinants of Child Growth in the First Two Years and Potential Interventions

Parul Christian

Department of International Health, Center for Human Nutrition, Bloomberg School of Public Health, The Johns Hopkins University, Baltimore, MD, USA

Abstract

In 2010, 171 million children under 5 years old were estimated to be stunted globally, with 98% being from low- and middle-income countries. Low birthweight including fetal growth restriction is also common in these regions and may contribute to childhood undernutrition. As part of the Child Health Reference Group (CHERG) and using 14 longitudinal birth cohorts and anthropometric measurements taken at 24 months of age, pooled odds ratios (ORs) were calculated to examine the relationship between small for gestational age (SGA) and preterm birth and subsequent stunting and wasting in children. Relative to term adequate size for gestational age (AGA), the OR (95% confidence interval) for stunting associated with AGA-preterm, SGA-term and SGA-preterm was 1.94 (1.59–2.36), 2.82 (2.40–3.32) and 4.98 (3.79–6.55), respectively. A similar magnitude of risk was also observed for wasting and underweight. This analysis indicates that childhood undernutrition may have its origins, in part, in the fetal period, suggesting a need to intervene during an earlier life stage during pregnancy and even preconceptionally, but also putting emphasis on maternal nutrition in general and adolescent nutrition. Interventions shown to impact fetal growth include antenatal supplementation with balanced calorie and protein, iron-folic acid, and multiple micronutrients. Nutrition-sensitive interventions such as delaying the first pregnancy, antimalarials and smoking cessation in some settings may be important.   © 2014 Nestec Ltd., Vevey/S. Karger AG, Basel

Background: Fetal Growth Restriction and Childhood Undernutrition

Although much progress has been made in the last two decades, 171 million pre-school children were estimated to be stunted globally in 2010, with 167.5 million from low- and middle-income countries (LMIC) [1]. This represents a prevalence of 26.7%, down from 39.7% in 1990. Secular trends in child stunting from 1990 to 2020 by region show significant progress in Asia, and continued improvements in Latin America but not in Africa, where a limited decline in stunting prevalence is recorded.

In LMIC, factors that influence linear growth in the first 2 years of life, the period during which growth faltering is found to be rapid, include: inappropriate breastfeeding and infant and young child feeding practices, i.e. inadequate frequency, quality and type of complementary foods; high incidence of infections including diarrheal morbidity [2]; a subclinical but ubiquitous condition in many settings such as environmental enteropathy [3], and mycotoxin exposures [4]. Postnatal interventions in the first 2 years of life that can have an impact include promotion of exclusive breastfeeding in the first 6 months of life and appropriate complementary feeding and other infant and young child feeding practices [5]. Integrated management of childhood illnesses may also impact stunting [6].

The recent focus on the first 1,000 days of life which includes the prenatal period draws attention to the need for intervening earlier in life, including during the critical period of fetal growth. Birthweight is a cumulative measure of intrauterine growth and gestational age. It is a commonly measured indicator of newborn health and is one of the leading factors influencing subsequent health and survival in many LMIC. Prevalence of low birthweight (LBW; <2,500 g) and its two contributory causes especially fetal growth restriction assessed using small for gestational age (SGA; defined as weight below the 10th percentile of a fetal growth reference for a given gestational age) continues to be high in LMIC [7]. The prevalence of LBW in 2010 is estimated to be 15%, whereas SGA is almost double of this at 27%, and may be as high as almost 45% in South Asia. The prevalence of preterm birth (gestational age <37 weeks) in LMIC is 11.4%. The three conditions may be discrete or have an overlap. In this example (fig. 1) [Christian et al., unpubl.] from rural Nepal, with prevalence of LBW, SGA, and preterm birth being 38.8, 55.4 and 21.2%, respectively, this overlap is seen, but there is still a considerable proportion of babies that are not LBW or preterm but are SGA. To note, the risk factors of SGA and preterm birth, and interventions to reduce these conditions are somewhat distinct. It is well recognized that SGA is a major cause of LBW in LMIC, unlike in high-income countries where preterm birth is more commonly an underlying biologic cause. High rates of LBW

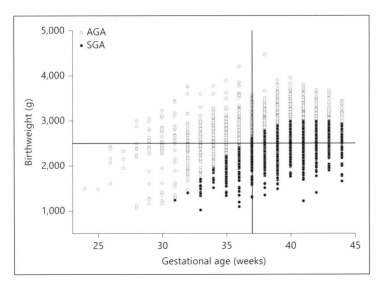

Fig. 1. Scatter plot of birthweight, gestation age, and SGA in rural southern Nepal. Christian et al. [unpubl.].

and childhood stunting coexist in many populations [8], indicating that small size at birth continues to track in the first 2 years of life. However, on average length-for-age z score of children at birth is closer to 0 to –0.5, which rapidly decreases to as low as –1.75 to –2.0 z score by 24 months of age, implicating postnatal rather than prenatal factors in causing this dramatic growth faltering. Still, studies linking birthweight and childhood undernutrition show a strong association [9], suggesting that growth in the first 1,000 days is better viewed as a continuum, but few analyses have examined systematically the contributions of fetal growth to childhood undernutrition.

Association between SGA, Preterm Birth and Child Undernutrition

As part of the Child Health Epidemiology Reference Group (www.cherg.org), we examined the contribution of fetal growth and preterm birth to childhood undernutrition in LMIC [10]. An extensive search of the existing literature was first undertaken to identify potential studies from LMIC that had collected prospective data on child (12–60 months of age) anthropometry in existing birth cohorts in which valid measurements of birthweight and gestational age were taken. In eligible cohorts, investigators were invited to provide data on birthweight, gestational age and child anthropometry. In a subgroup of these studies, child anthropometry was measured at 24 months of age. A total of 14 studies had

Table 1. Estimated risk for childhood undernutrition at 24 months of age by preterm birth, SGA and LBW categories in LMIC

	Preterm		SGA		LBW	
	OR	95% CI	OR	95% CI	OR	95% CI
Stunting	1.65	1.42–1.91	2.68	2.30–3.14	3.11	2.72–3.57
Wasting	1.35	1.06–1.72	2.42	1.89–3.11	3.13	2.21–4.43
Underweight	1.61	1.27–2.05	3.06	2.46–3.80	3.8	2.99–4.82

Stunting defined as length-for-age <–2 z score. Wasting defined as weight-for-length <–2 z score. Underweight defined as weight-for-age <–2 z score.

taken measurements on children (n = 18,061) and were analyzed to examine outcomes of stunting (length-for-age <–2 z), wasting (weight-for-length <–2 z), and underweight (weight-for-age <–2 z) at 24 months of age (table 1). Thus, this analysis represents a subset of that undertaken for children between 12 and 60 months of age [10].

SGA was defined as less than the 10th percentile for gestational age using the US population-based standard for fetal growth by Alexander et al. [11]. Precalculated odds ratios (ORs) and standard errors/confidence intervals from each study were used to derive regional and global estimates using meta-analysis with random-effects models. Between-study heterogeneity was quantified using the I^2 statistic (expressed as %) and Cochrane's Q (significance level <0.05). Forest plots were used to display pooled regional estimates. Analysis was done also by adjusting for child's age, sex, multiple gestation, infection, intervention, and mother's parity, socioeconomic status, education, infection and intervention, in data sets for which data were provided.

Figures 2 and 3 illustrate the ORs for stunting and wasting in children 24 months of age by categories of risk. Relative to adequate size for gestational age (AGA)-term birth, the ORs (95% CI) for stunting associated with AGA-preterm, SGA-term, and SGA-preterm were 1.94 (1.59, 2.36), 2.82 (2.40, 3.32) and 4.98 (3.79, 6.55), respectively, suggesting an additive risk in the presence of both conditions. A similar magnitude of risk was also observed for wasting and underweight (data not shown) among children. Preterm alone conferred a lower risk for stunting and the ORs were not statistically significant for wasting except in Latin America (fig. 3). Adjusted analyses showed limited attenuation of the ORs, indicating that confounding was unlikely to be a concern in this analysis. When the risk relationship was compared between those born SGA with normal birthweight and those who were born LBW and SGA, a dose-response relationship became evident; being born both LBW and SGA carried a higher risk

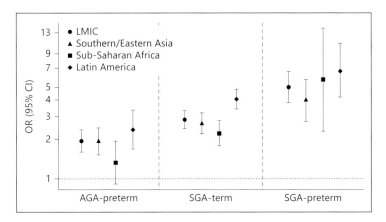

Fig. 2. Regional and overall ORs for childhood stunting at 24 months of age by size for gestational age and preterm and term birth combinations. Reference group is children born AGA and term.

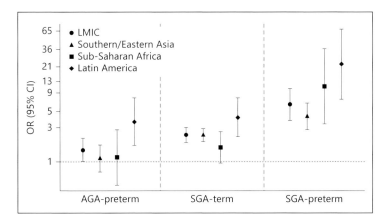

Fig. 3. Regional and overall ORs for childhood wasting at 24 months of age by size for gestational age and preterm and term birth combinations. Reference group is children born AGA and term.

(OR: 3.07, 95% CI: 2.32–4.08) than being SGA alone (OR: 1.91, 95% CI: 1.60–2.28).

This analysis reveals that childhood undernutrition, both stunting and wasting, may have its origins in the fetal period. Because fetal growth is strongly influenced by prepregnancy BMI and height, this analysis also shows that childhood undernutrition is related to maternal undernutrition prior to pregnancy. Despite the large variation in the prevalence of both SGA and preterm birth by region and country, the ORs of undernutrition associated with these exposures appeared to be quite comparable between regions, indicative of common underlying causes for fetal growth restriction and preterm birth. Latin America had the highest ORs, but the smaller sample sizes and lower prevalence of exposures in the studies from this region yielded more imprecise estimates of risk. As has been shown in other settings, the prevalence of SGA is higher than LBW. Strikingly, the coexistence of both preterm and SGA was remarkably low in many settings (1–2%). It has been shown that the etiologies of these conditions differ [12]. In addition, the lower prevalence of the two conditions combined was examined only in the surviving cohort of 24-month-olds, and the risk of mortality is shown to be highest in the group with both SGA and preterm [13]. Preterm-only babies have a lower probability of experiencing fetal growth restriction. One consideration is that the shorter time in utero, especially closer to term, may result in a lower risk of SGA among these babies.

Maternal Nutrition and Fetal Growth

Kramer [12] demonstrated over two decades ago that maternal nutritional factors account for more than 50% of the etiology of LBW in low-income countries. These factors included low prepregnancy weight, short stature, and low caloric intake during pregnancy or inadequate weight gain as well as maternal LBW itself, suggesting an intergenerational effect. Using data from a WHO collaborative study which included over 100,000 women, every 1 cm decrease in prepregnancy height or 1 unit decrease in prepregnancy BMI was associated with a 2-fold increased odds of intrauterine growth restriction [14]. Using cross-sectional data from 109 Demographic Health Surveys conducted between 1991 and 2008 in 54 developing countries and covering 2.6 million children aged 0–59 months, Özaltin et al. [15] showed that maternal height was inversely associated with risks of underweight, stunting, and wasting and child mortality. Compared with maternal height of >160 cm, those with height <145 cm had a 2-fold higher risk of their child being stunted. This is suggestive that the association of maternal stature with childhood nutritional status is mediated by the influence of maternal height on intrauterine growth [16]. While maternal height represents the culmination of environmental exposures from fetal to adulthood, including nutritional, infectious, lifestyle factors, and pregnancy in early adolescence, prepregnancy maternal BMI is more likely to capture aspects of short-term food availability, access to health care and other concurrent socioeconomic and cultural conditions at the onset of pregnancy.

Maternal short stature (<145 cm) continues to be high in many settings especially in South Asia [9]. Data from 54 demographic health studies that examined height among women 25–49 years of age from 1994 to 2008 revealed a wealth differential in the patterns of increase in mean height. In 35 of the countries, there was either a decline or stagnation in height among women, largely in the poorest wealth quintiles [17]. In many settings, early marriage leading to early pregnancies may impact adolescent nutritional status and growth. In a rural setting in northeastern Bangladesh, pregnancy in adolescence hampered linear and ponderal growth [18]. In this prospective cohort study, 162 adolescents in their first pregnancy were matched with 385 never-pregnant girls of the same achieved age and age since menarche. Annual growth in terms of height, weight, and mid-upper arm circumference, and percent body fat was significantly lower among pregnant girls compared to girls who did not become pregnant after adjusting for confounders. In fact, growth in height ceased in the pregnant girls, whereas the nonpregnant girls gained in height by 0.3 (SD = 0.8) cm over the course of the year-long follow-up. An estimated overall attained height loss ranging between 0.6 and 2.7 cm may have resulted from cessation of linear growth in adolescence due to an early pregnancy, which may be one contributory factor leading to adulthood stunting in women. Childbearing during the growth period from menarche through the teenage years is also associated with adverse birth outcomes such as premature birth and LBW. Potential strategies to prevent early pregnancy including incentives, legislation, availability of contraception, and registration of newly married may be important in many LMIC settings [19].

Potential Nutritional and Nonnutritional Interventions

Nutritional interventions during pregnancy have been shown to be beneficial for fetal growth as summarized by Ramakrishnan et al. [this vol., pp. 71–80]. Meta-analysis of trials of food (calorie and protein) supplementation during pregnancy has shown a reduction of 34% in the risk of SGA (RR: 0.68, 95% CI: 0.51–0.92) [20]. Daily iron folic acid and prenatal multiple micronutrient supplementation (without food) also shows a significant reduction in LBW with RR of 0.80 (95% CI: 0.71–0.90) [21], and in SGA with RR 0.83 (95% CI: 0.73–0.95), respectively [22]. Although routine iron-folic acid supplement use, despite widespread policy in many countries continues to be low [23], combining food and micronutrient intervention approaches in settings with maternal undernutrition and micronutrient deficiencies would help address the high burden of fetal growth restriction, and in addition yield better nutritional status in the offspring. Although evidence is limited [24], cash transfer or food vouchers for women during pregnancy in food-insecure settings may be beneficial and should be tested for their impact on birthweight and fetal growth. Examples of food transfer systems are available from programs in India, Nigeria and Ethiopia [19]. Very few nutritional interventions have enhanced gestational length of a pregnancy or shown to reduce preterm birth, except perhaps for prenatal zinc [25] or calcium supplementation [26].

Although not nutritional, certain lifestyle interventions may be important for alleviating the burden of fetal growth restriction and preterm birth. For example, tobacco smoking is a well-known risk factor sharing a dose-response relationship with both the occurrence of LBW and preterm delivery. After adjusting for confounders, passive smoking is also known to elevate the risk of fetal growth restriction. Interventions targeted at smoking cessation can be effective in reducing adverse birth outcomes. A systematic Cochrane meta-analysis that included 72 trials, both individual and cluster-randomized, has shown reductions in smoking during pregnancy and in outcomes of LBW (RR: 0.83, 95% CI: 0.73–0.95) and preterm birth (RR: 0.86, 95% CI: 0.74–0.98) [27]. Globally, reproductive/urinary tract infections, HIV-1, and malaria may be the largest infectious causes of LBW and preterm. In malarious settings, the new WHO recommendation is to provide at least 3 doses of SP (sulfadoxine-pyrimethamine) during pregnancy. Seven trials comparing 3 or more versus 2 doses of SP did better in reducing placental malaria, and also in reducing mild to moderate anemia by 40% and LBW by 20% (RR: 0.80, 95% CI: 0.69–0.94) [28]. Bacterial vaginosis (BV) is also known to increase the risk of preterm birth. Asymptomatic BV is associated with a 2-fold increased risk of preterm birth, or nearly 3-fold when BV is detected prior to 16 weeks of gestation [29]. In a meta-analysis of 15 small trials, BV treatment during pregnancy resulted in no overall impact on risk of preterm birth, except among women treated before 20 weeks of gestation (OR: 0.63, 95% CI: 0.48–0.84) [30]. Interventions to reduce indoor air pollution seem promising. Exposure to pollution from solid fuel compared with cleaner fuels or stoves with chimneys has shown to significantly increase the risk of LBW and preterm birth by 38% (OR: 1.38, 95% CI: 1.25–1.52) [31]. In many LMIC, outdoor and vehicular air pollution especially in urban areas may be high and on the rise, and interventions for ameliorating their adverse effects need testing. Although deworming twice during pregnancy when provided as a service in a research setting was found to significantly reduce maternal anemia, severe anemia, LBW and infant mortality [32], the evidence from randomized controlled trials is lacking [33].

Beyond periconceptional folic acid use shown to reduce the risk of neural tube defects, there is limited evidence from rigorous randomized controlled trials to show the impact of pre- or periconceptional nutritional interventions on birth outcomes. Although numerous observational studies link maternal nutritional status, especially low prepregnancy maternal BMI and height, with outcomes of fetal growth restriction, and to some extent with preterm birth, confounding may be a serious problem. There is a need to conduct large trials of preconception nutritional supplementation in settings with high rates of maternal undernutrition and fetal growth restriction [34].

Conclusion

The burden of child undernutrition continues to be high in many LMIC. The intergenerational cycle of growth failure exists in many of these settings, with coexisting high burdens of maternal undernutrition including short stature, fetal growth restriction, and childhood stunting. In industrialized settings and in wealthy households in LMIC, average maternal height has shown a systematic increase over time, in contrast to stagnating in underresourced, poorer households, suggesting that environmental influences could lead to improvements over time. The analysis linking SGA to risk of stunting and wasting in childhood provides further impetus for a life course approach for interventions as reflected in the emphasis on the first 1,000 days. Numerous prenatal interventions have shown to be effective in improving fetal growth and size at birth, including iron-folic acid that is policy in many areas of the world, as well as multiple micronutrient, and food/energy-protein supplementation in food-insecure conditions. In addition, the nutrition and health state of a woman when she conceives sets the stage for the well-being of the pregnancy and the trajectory of the growth and development of her fetus, suggesting that preconceptional and early-pregnancy interventions may be important, but data on impact are limited. There is an urgent need for future research to examine the additional benefit of pre- and periconceptional macro- and micronutrient interventions in enhancing birth outcomes, especially fetal growth and gestational duration. Focusing on an equally important life stage of adolescence may yield improvements in reproductive health outcomes, while at the same time enhancing the linear growth and nutritional status of girls. Delaying a first pregnancy could be a powerful intervention in this respect.

In conclusion, policy and programmatic focus on maternal nutrition and health are central for combating the large burden of fetal and childhood undernutrition as we evaluate progress towards the MDGs and develop future strategies.

Acknowledgement

The analysis on fetal growth, preterm birth and child undernutrition was undertaken as part of a CHERG activity. The group that contributed to this work include Sun Eun Lee, Moira Donahue Angel, Linda S. Adair, Shams E. Arifeen, Per Ashorn, Fernando C. Barros, Caroline H.D. Fall, Wafaie W. Fawzi, Wei Hao, Gang Hu, Jean H. Humphrey, Lieven Huybregts, Charu V. Joglekar, Simon K. Kariuki, Patrick Kolsteren, Ghattu V. Krishnaveni, Enqing Liu, Reynaldo Martorell, David Osrin, Lars-Ake Persson, Usha Ramakrishnan, Linda Richter, Dominique Roberfroid, Ayesha Sania, Feiko O. Ter Kuile, James Tielsch, Cesar G. Victora, Chittaranjan S. Yajnik, Hong Yan, Lingxia Zeng, Robert E. Black. The analysis was supported by the Bill and Melinda Gates Foundation, Seattle, Wash., USA.

Disclosure Statement

The author has no conflicts of interest to declare.

References

1 de Onis M, Blossner M, Borghi E: Prevalence and trends of stunting among preschool children, 1990–2020. Pub Health Nutr 2012;15: 142–148.
2 Checkley W, Buckley G, Gilman RH, et al: Multi-country analysis of the effects of diarrhoea on childhood stunting. Int J Epidemiol 2008;37:816–830.
3 Prendergast A, Kelly P: Enteropathies in the developing world: neglected effects on global health. Am J Trop Med Hyg 2012;86:756–763.
4 Smith LE, Stoltzfus RJ, Prendergast A: Food chain mycotoxin exposure, gut health, and impaired growth: a conceptual framework. Adv Nutr 2012;3:526–531.
5 Bhutta ZA, Ahmed T, Black RE, et al: What works? Interventions for maternal and child undernutrition and survival. Lancet 2008; 371:417–440.
6 Arifeen SE, Hoque DM, Akter T, et al: Effect of the integrated management of childhood illness strategy on childhood mortality and nutrition in a rural area in Bangladesh: a cluster randomised trial. Lancet 2009;374:393–403.
7 Lee AC, Katz J, Blencowe H, et al, the CHERG IUGR-Preterm Working Group: Born too small: national estimates of term and preterm small-for-gestational-age in low-middle income countries in 2010. Lancet Global Health 2013, in press.
8 United Nations, Subcommittee on Nutrition: Third report on the world nutrition situation: a report compiled from information available to the ACC/SCN. Geneva, United Nations, 1997.
9 Christian P: Prenatal origins of malnutrition; in Kalhan S, Prentice A, Yajnik C (eds): Emerging Societies: Co-Existence of Childhood Malnutrition and Obesity. Nestle Nutr Inst Workshop Ser Pediatr Program. Vevey, Nestec/Basel, Karger, vol 63, 2009.
10 Christian P, Lee SE, Donahue MA, et al: Risk of childhood undernutrition related to small-for-gestational age and preterm birth in low and middle income countries. Int J Epi 2013, E-pub ahead of print.
11 Alexander GR, Himes JH, Kaufman RB, et al: A United States national reference for fetal growth. Obstet Gynecol 1996;87:163–168.
12 Kramer MS: Intrauterine growth and gestational duration determinants. Pediatrics 1987;80:502–511.
13 Katz J, Lee ACC, Kozuki N, et al, the CHERG Intrauterine Growth Restriction-Preterm Birth Working Group: Mortality risk in preterm and small-for-gestational-age infants in low-income and middle-income countries: a pooled country analysis. Lancet 2013;382: 417–425.
14 Ramakrishnan U: Nutrition and low birth weight: from research to practice. Am J Clin Nutr 2004;79:17–21.
15 Özaltin E, Hill K, Subramanian SV: Association of maternal stature with offspring mortality, underweight, and stunting in low- to middle-income countries. JAMA 2010;303: 1507–1516.
16 Christian P: Maternal height and risk of child mortality and undernutrition (editorial). JAMA 2010;303:1539–1549.

17 Subramanian SV, Özaltin E, Finlay JE: Height of nations: a socioeconomic analysis of cohort differences and patterns among women in 54 low- to middle-income countries. PLoS One 2011;6:e18962.

18 Rah JH, Christian P, Shamim AA, et al: Pregnancy and lactation hinder growth and nutritional status of adolescent girls in rural Bangladesh. J Nutr 2008;138:1505–1511.

19 Mason JB, Saldanha LS, Ramakrishnan U, et al: Opportunities for improving maternal nutrition and birth outcomes: synthesis of country experiences. Food Nutr Bull 2012; 33(suppl 2):S104–S137.

20 Imdad A, Bhutta ZA: Maternal nutrition and birth outcomes. Effect of balanced protein-energy supplementation. Paediatr Perinat Epidemiol 2012;26(suppl 1):178–190.

21 Imdad A, Bhutta ZA: Routine iron/folate supplementation during pregnancy: effect on maternal anaemia and birth outcomes. Paediatr Perinat Epidemiol 2012;26(suppl 1):168–177.

22 Ramakrishnan U, Grant FK, Goldenberg T, et al: Effect of multiple micronutrient supplementation on pregnancy and infant outcomes: a systematic review. Paediatr Perinat Epidemiol 2012;26(suppl 1):153–167.

23 Christian P: Nutrition and maternal mortality in developing countries; in Lammi-Keefe CJ, Couch S, Philipson E (eds): Handbook of Nutrition and Pregnancy. Totowa, Humana Press, 2008.

24 Barber SL, Gertler PJ: The impact of Mexico's conditional cash transfer programme, Oportunidades, on birthweight. Trop Med Int Heal 2008;13:1405–1414.

25 Chaffee BW, King JC: Effect of zinc supplementation on pregnancy and infant outcomes: a systematic review. Paediatr Perinat Epidemiol 2012;26(suppl):118–137.

26 Imdad A, Bhutta ZA: Effects of calcium supplementation during pregnancy on maternal, fetal and birth outcomes. Paediatr Perinat Epidemiol 2012;26(suppl):138–152.

27 Lumley J, Chamberlain C, Dowswell T, et al: Interventions for promoting smoking cessation during pregnancy. Cochrane Database Syst Rev 2009;CD001055.

28 Kayentao K, Garner P, van Eijk AM: Intermittent preventive therapy for malaria during pregnancy using 2 vs. 3 or more doses of sulfadoxine-pyrimethamine and risk of low birth weight in Africa: systematic review and meta-analysis. JAMA 2013;309:594–604.

29 Leitich H, Kiss H: Asymptomatic bacterial vaginosis and intermediate flora as risk factors for adverse pregnancy outcome. Best Pract Res Clin Obstet Gynaecol 2007;21:375–390.

30 McDonald HM, Brocklehurst P, Gordon A: Antibiotics for treating bacterial vaginosis in pregnancy. Cochrane Database Syst Rev 2007;CD000262.

31 Pope DP, Mishra V, Thompson L, et al: Risk of low birth weight and stillbirth associated with indoor air pollution from solid fuel use in developing countries. Epidemiol Rv 2010; 32:70–81.

32 Christian P, Khatry SK, West KP Jr: Antenatal anthelminthic therapy, birth weight and infant survival in rural Nepal. Lancet 2004; 364:981–983.

33 Imhoff-Kunsch B, Briggs V: Antihelminthics in pregnancy and maternal, newborn and child health. Paediatr Perinat Epidemiol 2012;26(suppl):223–238.

34 Ramakrishnan U, Grant F, Goldenberg T, et al: Effect of women's nutrition before and during early pregnancy on maternal and infant outcomes: a systematic review. Paediatr Perinat Epidemiol 2012;26(suppl 1):285–301.

Evidence on Interventions and Field Experiences

Black RE, Singhal A, Uauy R (eds): International Nutrition: Achieving Millennium Goals and Beyond.
Nestlé Nutr Inst Workshop Ser, vol 78, pp 93–109, (DOI: 10.1159/000354946)
Nestec Ltd., Vevey/S. Karger AG., Basel, © 2014

How Can Agricultural Interventions Contribute in Improving Nutrition Health and Achieving the MDGs in Least-Developed Countries?

Andrew Dorward

SOAS, University of London, and Leverhulme Center for Integrative Research in Agriculture and Health, London, UK

Abstract

There are strong conceptual linkages between agricultural development and nutrition improvements which may be categorized into three main pathways: the development, own-production and market pathways. Evidence on the efficacy of these pathways is mixed with some strong, some negative and some weak impacts. These findings reflect both the importance of agriculture for nutrition and the conditionality of that importance on contextual factors. They are also the result of insufficient high-quality empirical research investigating these linkages. The most effective 'pathways' and interventions linking agricultural change to improved nutritional outcomes change with economic growth and development, with declining importance of the development and own-production pathways and increasing importance of the market pathway. Substantial challenges in operationalizing agricultural-nutrition linkages need to be overcome to better exploit potential opportunities.   © 2014 Nestec Ltd., Vevey/S. Karger AG, Basel

Introduction

This chapter discusses ways in which agricultural interventions can contribute to improving nutrition health and to achieving the Millennium Development Goals (MDGs) in least-developed countries. After this introduction, the chapter briefly details the main nutrition- and agriculture-related MDGs and progress on their achievement. The following section then considers processes by which agriculture may contribute to improved nutrition and to progress on nutrition-related MDGs. This is followed by an examination of evidence on the impact of agricultural development and development interventions on nutrition. This leads on to a discussion of agricultural interventions that can promote improved nutrition – sometimes referred to as nutrition-sensitive agriculture.

What Are the Nutrition/Health Issues in the MDGs That Are Most Closely Linked to Agriculture?

The MDGs, a set of eight goals with associated targets and indicators, were originally specified in United Nations [1]. A small number of further targets and indicators were added subsequently.

The principle goal and target that is the focus of this paper is Goal 1 (eradicate extreme poverty and hunger) and within that target 1C (halve, between 1990 and 2015, the proportion of people who suffer from hunger). Two indicators are specified for this target:
- Indicator 1.8: prevalence of underweight children younger than 5 years
- Indicator 1.9: proportion of population below minimum level of dietary energy consumption

The most recent information on progress and likely achievement or non-achievement of MDG targets is found in United Nations [2]. Substantial gains have been made on indicator 1.8 in some regions (notably Western Asia, Eastern Asia, Caucasus and Central Asia and Latin America and the Caribbean, and to a lesser extent in North Africa and South Eastern Asia). However, progress has been slower in Sub-Saharan Africa and South Asia, and the overall target of halving the prevalence of under-nourishment is unlikely to be met by 2015.[1]

There have been considerable concerns about the validity of measures for indicators used for indicator 1.9. Revised estimates of the numbers and proportions of undernourished people are provided in [5]. These show that prior to 2007, falls in the prevalence of undernourished people were not quite on track to meet the MDG target, and food price increases in 2008 and subsequent years then further slowed down the rate of fall in incidence. However, absolute numbers of undernourished people have hardly fallen, meaning that the World Food Summit global target of halving the number of hungry people from 1990–1992

---

[1] This discussion of MDG achievements does not address widely voiced concerns about differences between changes in incidence and absolute numbers or about greater challenges in meeting relative rather than absolute reductions where countries or regions have initially high incidences of disadvantage [3].

to 2015 will be missed by a wide margin. However, the revised estimates of prevalence of undernourishment show a decline rather than the previously estimated reversal in falling global prevalence of undernourishment following food price rises in 2008, as also reported by Headey [4].

As with other MDG targets, there are wide variations between regions as regards changes in prevalence and numbers of undernourished people. FAO, WFP and IFAD [5] estimate that absolute numbers of undernourished people have been falling in Asia and in the Latin America-Caribbean areas, with falls in prevalence on track to meet the MDG target. In both Near East/North Africa and Sub-Saharan Africa, however, absolute numbers of undernourished people have been rising, with lower falls in prevalence in Sub-Saharan Africa, but actual increases in prevalence in Near East and North Africa – although this is from a much lower 1990–1992 starting point than the other regions (7% as compared with 15% in Latin America/Caribbean, 25% in Asia and 35% in Sub-Saharan Africa). Within Asia, there has been a remarkable fall in prevalence in South Eastern Asia from 30 to 11% from 1990–1992 to 2010, with a slightly lower but still remarkable fall in Eastern Asia from 21 to 12% over the same period. South Asia achieved a lower fall in prevalence, however, which if continued will not be enough to achieve the target. Prevalence in Western Asia increased.

FAO, WFP and IFAD [5] recommend that although undernourishment and hunger should be monitored with a wide range of indicators of food availability, access and utilization, data are not available on an annual regional basis for many critical indicators, such as stunting and wasting.

How Can Agriculture Contribute to Improvements in Nutrition?

Links between agriculture and food security have long been recognized, but agriculture is only one contributor to food security. The Committee on World Food Security defines food security as follows [6]:

Food security exists when all people, at all times, have physical, social and economic access to sufficient, safe and nutritious food that meets their dietary needs and food preferences for an active and healthy life. The four pillars of food security are availability, access, utilization and stability. The nutritional dimension is integral to the concept of food security.

This recognizes that food availability is a necessary but not sufficient condition for food security – access is also necessary through entitlements (allowing local unavailability to be overcome by purchases), and once accessed food needs to be utilized. Utilization depends upon food storage and processing and upon physiological processes of nutrient absorption. Stability is then needed in expected food access – and hence stability in availability, access and utilization and in their determinants. Food security also has different dimensions as regards types of nutrient.

A number of authors have provided overviews and conceptualizations of links between agriculture and nutrition or, more widely, health [7–12]. It is helpful to distinguish between three broad pathways by which agriculture impacts on nutrition: a general development pathway, a market pathway, and an own-production pathway.[2] We consider these in turn.

There is a longstanding literature on the role of agricultural development in wider development processes [14–16] supported by more recent empirical work [17]. This may be summarized as a process whereby new agricultural technologies and resources increase both agricultural production and food availability per worker [18]. This lowers the cost and price of food relative to worker incomes and increases real incomes and other discretionary spending. It also releases agricultural labor from food production to production of other goods and services. Industrial, service and knowledge revolutions can then build on this with further increases in labor productivity and in goods and services supply and demand, with falling relative importance of agriculture. Expected food security and nutritional benefits from this arise from increased food production (improving food availability), lower food prices and increased real incomes (improving food access, both for staples and more diverse nutrient rich foods) and more diverse incomes (improving food stability). Increased individual and public incomes should also lead to improved individual and public educational, health, sanitation and other investments which should lead to improved food utilization. These development processes should therefore lead to improvements in all four 'pillars' of food security.

These arguments suggest that despite its challenges there is a special role for smallholder agricultural development in poor agrarian economies with large numbers of poor farmers: such development leads to simultaneous expansion of labor supply to and demand for initially nonstaple and then nonfarm production with simultaneous food security and nutritional gains for poor smallholder populations. The effectiveness and efficiency of smallholder development policies and investments are, however, questioned by some, who suggest that faster growth may be achieved by focusing on nonagricultural growth and/or large-scale agricultural development [19]. These arguments rely on prior or current agricultural development that has already raised agricultural productivity outside the poor agrarian economy to deliver cheap food (from imports or from

[2] This builds on the distinction between market and own-production pathways [13] and on four out of five pathways identified in World Bank [12].

rapid increases in net value-added labor productivity in large-scale agricultural development) with simultaneous nonagricultural development to absorb small-holder labor and raise its productivity outside the agricultural sector. This in turn requires competitive access to markets serving populations with sufficiently high incomes to demand the new goods and services produced. Both these alternatives face substantial challenges as regards large-scale requirements for improved access to food markets and for labor-absorbing nonagricultural development. Large-scale social protection policies may address some of these challenges (as in Brazil) as policy makers try to produce the same coordinated processes with taxes and subsidies transferring income to large numbers of poor rural people from smaller numbers of skilled workers and owners of capital. This approach, however, faces governance and political economy challenges and needs a large and rapidly growing capital-intensive sector to support these transfers.

There are also questions about the availability of cheap food. International food price spikes from 2008 have led to renewed interest in food prices and challenged the widespread observation of a steady fall in long-term real food prices [20]. Prices have subsequently fluctuated above a base somewhat higher than pre-2008 prices. More fundamentally, however, conventional measures of 'real' food prices compare food prices with US consumer prices or the prices of manufactures, prices that are largely determined in richer economies by the demand of richer consumers and societies (with relative falls in food prices an inevitable result of increasing incomes with economic growth [18, 21]). A more meaningful measure of real food prices is to compare them with incomes, which vary between rich and poor individuals and societies. Unsurprisingly, real international food prices measured in this way have not declined for poor people in the way that they have for the less poor [18].

The market and own-production pathways are shown in figure 1. Both these pathways postulate the effects of agricultural interventions (on the left) which, if taken up, lead to agricultural product changes. Under the market pathway (see the upper part of fig. 1), these product changes then lead to changes in the supply to the food market, with possible subsequent impacts on food prices, consumer real incomes and food demand and consumption, with possible subsequent impacts on nutrition intakes, food utilization and nutritional status. There are strong parallels between the market pathway and some of the processes outlined under the agricultural development pathway. However, the market pathway is not restricted to economies with large numbers of poor farmers, and focusses more on impacts on the nutrition of food buyers.

The own-production pathway (in the lower part of fig. 1) focusses more on food consumption and nutritional status impacts for agricultural producers –

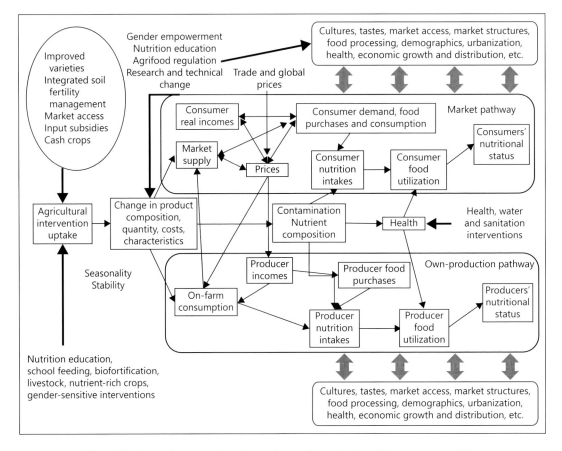

Fig. 1. Market and own-production pathways for agricultural impacts on nutrition.

allowing for the effects of increased incomes from food or nonfood sales and/or own changes in consumption of own-produced foods. Both pathways are affected by wider socioeconomic context (shown at the top and bottom of fig. 1) and by impacts of health, water and sanitation interventions (in the middle of fig. 1).

This discussion may appear to suggest that these three pathways can be considered relatively distinct from each other. There are, however, considerable overlaps between them – for example the development pathway depends upon processes that are very similar to those involved in the market pathway, and there are also linkages between the market and own-production pathways. The pathways are therefore both distinct and overlapping, as shown in figure 2 (which also shows important nonagricultural and contextual influences on nutritional status).

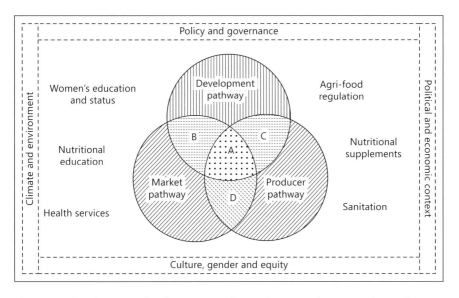

Fig. 2. Overlaps between development, market and own-production pathways for agricultural impacts on nutrition.

How Has Agriculture Contributed to Improvements in Nutrition?

We now consider evidence for agriculture's actual impacts on nutrition through these three pathways. As one would expect, there are considerable overlaps in evidence across the three pathways, but also considerable gaps and difficulties in clearly establishing patterns of causality.

Evidence on the first pathway is derived from two main types of study: those that analyze patterns of change across countries with different growth paths [9, 22], and those that look at growth paths in more detail within particular countries [23, 24]. Evenson and Gollin [25] also use a simulation approach to investigate the impact of the green revolution food production, prices and malnutrition.

A number of recent studies have investigated the relationship between income growth and nutrition, generally measured in terms of stunting, height-for-age or underweight [7, 9, 22, 23]. These generally find that increasing income leads to reduced malnutrition, although estimates of the strength of the relationship vary. Some studies provide some explanation of this variation, with stronger effects in longer-term analysis, from agricultural growth (except in India), and at lower income levels. Effects are also commonly stronger when malnutrition is measured by hunger or dietary intake than when it is measured by anthropometric variables. Nutritional status is also affected by the type of agriculture and by a range of conditioning factors including women's education and status, distribution of growth, dietary quality, land distribution, access to medical care, fertility, infrastructure, and specific nutrition programs. Headey [9] concludes that 'economic growth is nutrition-sensitive if it increases food production (especially when food insecurity is high), reduces poverty, increases female education, improves health access, and reduces fertility rates (…) for low-income countries at least, economic growth is a necessary but insufficient condition for reducing malnutrition'.

Data and estimation difficulties and the many influences on growth impacts on malnutrition mean that estimates of the scale of these impacts should be treated with care. It is nevertheless instructive to note the scale of the different estimates of an author who considers in some detail the variability and reliability in his estimates [9]. His regression estimates suggest that with a per capita growth rate of 5% per year, stunting prevalence would be reduced by around 0.9 percentage points per year. Outside India, agricultural growth per total capita of 5% per year would reduce stunting prevalence by 4 or 2 percentage points depending on the way that the sectors are weighted. No significant effect of agricultural growth on stunting prevalence is found in the Indian states. As regards impacts of agricultural growth on estimated calorie availability, a 5% increase in agricultural GDP per total capita leads to a 2.5–4% increase in energy supply, declining sharply as agricultural population shares fall and calorie consumption rises. A 10% increase in energy supply is then associated with a reduction in stunting of 3.3 percentage points. Increases in food production have similar impact for the group of countries with initial food production below the sample mean, but are very low and not significant for the group of countries with initial food production above the mean. Evenson and Gollin [25], using a simulation, estimate that without the Green Revolution the incidence of stunting would have been 12–15 percentage points higher in South Asia and 6–8 percentage points higher in developing countries overall.

The studies reported above are relevant to all three pathways by which agriculture can impact on nutrition – and emphasize the relationship and overlap between them. All three pathways can involve impacts from price changes and from changes in product composition, although the balance between them is likely to differ. There can also be significant complementarity, as between the development and own-production pathways, as the nutritional impacts of economic development tend to be greater in economies with greater relative importance of the agricultural sector. There is then a larger share of the workforce working in agriculture and getting a double benefit as both producers and consumers from increases in real incomes and in access to improved diets.

It is also useful, however, to distinguish between them:

- Market pathways generally involve more direct and immediate impacts of changes in food prices and food composition and less extensive processes of change. The development pathway, however, involves wider, medium- to long-term processes including effects of structural change, changes in agricultural and nonagricultural productivity, and impacts on individual and public resources and investments
- Development pathway impacts are more important in poorer, low- and middle-income countries, but market pathways can also be important in high-income countries

In the market pathway, we focus on two main mechanisms: changes in food prices and in food composition, noting first that if these changes are to be driven by changes in domestic agriculture, then this requires that food markets are not dominated by imports.

Some evidence on the impacts of short-term falls in food prices has been discussed earlier under the development pathway. Further evidence of short-term impacts is provided by examination of the negative impacts of food price rises. As discussed earlier, initial estimates of very large and damaging increases in the incidence of undernourishment and hunger following the 2008 global food price spike [26–28] have been moderated by the countervailing effects of economic growth benefiting poor people mainly in Asia [4, 5]. Medium-term damaging effects of higher food prices on the urban poor are universally recognized, but there is more debate on the effects of higher food prices on the rural poor. Some argue that the rural poor gain long-term benefits from higher food prices stimulating increased production and labor demand. Others, however, argue that the evidence for this is limited and that there are a number of structural constraints and considerations that make this unlikely for most poor rural people, particularly in Africa [29].

There is also some evidence of the negative effects of recent food price rises on nutritional status [28, 30]. Earlier studies of the effects of high rice prices also found increased malnutrition rates as a result of price rises in Indonesia and Bangladesh [31, 32]. Increases in rice prices may also lead to households reducing consumption of important micronutrients but not of calories as they try to maintain calorie consumption by reallocating spending to a less diverse diet with a higher proportion of staples.

Changes in dietary composition may result from changes in the mix of foods accessed by consumers or by changes in particular foods' nutrient composition as, for example, with the growth in the market demand for and consumption of orange flesh sweet potato and hence of vitamin A in rural Mozambique following its introduction to and cultivation by smallholder farmers [33, cited by 34]. 'Nutrition value chain' interventions have also promoted increased crop diversity in production and in consumer food intake, in both developing and developed economies [34].

Agricultural interventions' nutritional impacts via the own-production pathway have been the subject of a number of reviews [12, 35–37]. These draw similar conclusions, that the evidence base is too weak to draw any robust conclusions regarding the nutritional impacts on producers of the limited number of agricultural interventions investigated. Weaknesses in evidence arose as a result of poor study designs with limited counterfactuals, small sample sizes, and heterogeneous use of variables for measuring nutrition (including measures of dietary changes but relatively few measures of nutritional outcomes). However, all studies also report promising indications and examples of agricultural interventions impacting on nutritional status, and conclude that more and better quality studies are needed. It should be noted that these reviews did not cover agricultural interventions undertaken without specific nutritional objectives. Nevertheless, informative examples of such studies exist [38], and more systematic examination of them could be instructive.

In this context, a recent review identifies gaps in current and planned research on agriculture for nutrition [8]. Areas relevant to this paper and addressed by only a limited number of (or no) projects included: whole supply and nutrition impact chains and policy influences on them; the development pathway; the market pathway; governance, policy processes and political economy influences; cost-effectiveness, and development of research and evaluation methods and metrics. They did not, however, attempt to assess the quality of the research projects reviewed.

What Agricultural Interventions Can Promote Improved Nutrition Health and Achievement of the MDGs in Least Developed Countries?

In this section, we build on earlier discussion and the work of other authors to identify strategic principles, practical principles and practical options for 'nutrition-sensitive agriculture', agricultural interventions aiming to promote improved nutrition.

Discussion in the sections above shows that the effectiveness of agricultural development in promoting improved nutrition is generally highest in poorer agrarian economies, and declines with development, as does the proportion of agricultural workers and rural inhabitants. This suggests declining importance of the development and own-production pathways. The importance of the market pathway, on the other hand, increases with development, as food buyers and purchases increase and subsistence production and consumption decline. Referring back to figure 2, these patterns suggest that agri-nutrition interventions in the least developed, poor agrarian economies are likely to be most effective if they work in the overlap of the development and own-production pathways (intersection C). As development proceeds, the focus should shift towards areas A and D, before concentrating on the market pathway – although there will still be some disadvantaged producers who merit specific attention through own-production pathways, as well as poor consumers whose nutrition could benefit from some engagement in own production of particular foods (such as vegetables, fruit or small livestock). Agri-nutrition interventions will also need to be supported and complemented by other services and interventions and a supportive environment as shown in figure 2, particularly where there are substantial food imports. This pattern of changing pathways has parallels with changing roles for governments in promoting agriculture [39] (establishing the basics, kick starting markets, facilitating markets) and in promoting agricultural nutrition links [40], with provision of core public goods in stage one (energy- and nutrient-deficient) countries, targeted service delivery in stage two (energy-sufficient but nutrient-deficient) countries, and private sector regulation in stage three (excessive calorie) countries.

It must also be recognized that as important players in the value chain, producers' interests will be important in any intervention that seeks to change agricultural practices, even if improvement of their nutrition is not an objective driving that intervention.

These broad strategic principles are supported by and match more practical principles for nutrition-sensitive agriculture. Hawkes and Ruel [34] outline nine principles for what they term a 'nutrition value chain' approach – which has wider relevance beyond interventions within the market pathway (as almost all agricultural development involves markets, even if nutrition objectives are not pursued through food markets). The following principles are suggested [34, pp. 35–38]:

1   Start with explicit nutrition goals.
2   Clearly define the nutrition problem.
3   Create and capture value for nutrition.
4   Be expansive in the search for solutions, but tailor to context.
5   Focus on the functioning and coordination of the whole chain in order to create sustainable solutions.
6   Add value not only for nutrition (and consumers), but also for other chain actors.
7   Take a broader view of adding value for producers and consumers.
8   Focus on meeting, growing, and creating demand.
9   Create a policy environment in which better nutrition is valued.

Herforth et al. [41] also suggest principles for nutrition-sensitive agriculture, focusing on guiding principles for operational investments that prioritize nutrition in agriculture and rural development. They reiterate the first of Hawkes and Ruel's principles and suggest the targeting of nutritionally vulnerable groups, investment in women, and a focus on increasing all-year access to diverse, nutrient-dense foods. They also argue for creation of enabling environments for good nutrition through knowledge and incentives for staff, and active search for opportunities to work across sectors. These points demand active involvement of different specialists in agriculture, nutrition and other development sectors and new cross-sectoral thinking and disciplines to address these issues. World Bank [12] note the need for investment in human capacity and behavioral change alongside agricultural intervention if such interventions are to have nutritional impacts.

Fan et al. [42] set out wider principles for promoting beneficial linkages of both health and nutrition with agriculture. These focus on filling knowledge gaps (through research, evaluation and education across disciplines and sectors), doing no harm (addressing health risks along agricultural value chains right through to consumers and seeking to promote health and nutrition interventions that contribute to the productivity of agricultural labor), seeking out and scaling up innovative solutions in sectoral programs with cross-sectoral benefits, and creating an environment in which cooperation can thrive (through cross-sectoral partnerships with mutual accountability mechanisms, attention to market failures and advocacy). These are particularly useful in also emphasizing the importance of feedbacks from nutrition to agriculture and health: these feedbacks have not been a focus of this paper but are nevertheless important.

Finally, we consider practical options for nutrition-sensitive agriculture. Figure 1 includes some examples of the types of agricultural intervention that may be useful in nutrition sensitive agriculture. Hawkes and Ruel [34] also outline five 'categories of action' within the value chain approach they espouse: information and education for behavior change; research and technology change (for example through breeding, genetic modification, fertilization, or agronomy to increase production or change product composition); organizational change, within and among organizations, to promote coordination or change power relations; changes in costs and incentives (through new systems or public or private investments), and development of policies and standards (such as procurement policies and systems or market or food safety standards). To these might be added, from a wider perspective, changes in national policies (for example on trade, input or product subsidies).

We now briefly discuss food contamination, an issue spanning the market and own-production pathways in figure 1. We focus on mycotoxin contamination, specifically aflatoxin, which is produced by *Aspergillus flavus* and *A. parasiticus* infecting maize grain through insect attack in the field and/or in poor storage conditions. High concentrations of aflatoxin are found in maize in southern, eastern and west Africa as well as in parts of Asia and Latin America. Aflatoxins' effects in inducing liver cancer have long been recognized, but there is a growing body of evidence of immune system disorders and stunted growth with exposure to aflatoxin and fumonisin (another common mycotoxin). These effects are particularly important in poor populations where maize is a staple food often produced under stress and then stored in poor conditions (groundnuts, rice, dried cassava, and sorghum, and millet are also affected). They are also particularly serious in the first 1,000 days of life. Given the widespread poor storage and consumption of (particularly) maize and the high incidence of communicable diseases to which these mycotoxins may suppress immunity, this is a major issue with strong links between agriculture and nutrition. Possible measures include improved crop pest control, changes in storage practices to reduce insect infestation/damage and moisture content, infection of grain with competing and harmless fungal species, rejection of affected grain, mineral or yeast-based binder additives, and market standards and regulations. Interventions must however take account of the poverty and food insecurity of many affected households, the importance of dispersed and informal markets with small transactions in areas with very poor market infrastructure, and the importance of subsistence production and consumption which never enters the market [43–45].

Conclusions

This review has shown that achievement of the nutrition-related MDGs is unlikely in large populations of poor people mainly in South Asia and Sub-Saharan Africa, but that agricultural development can promote nutrition improvements through three main pathways (the development, own production and market pathways). Evidence on the efficacy of these pathways is mixed with some strong and some weak or negative impacts, reflecting varied processes and contexts as well as insufficient high-quality empirical research. It is clear, however, that there is significant potential for improving the nutritional status of poor people through a range of agricultural interventions alongside complementary social and nutritional interventions – with particular attention to the status of women.

We conclude with a brief discussion of the major challenges to implementing agricultural interventions to achieve improved nutrition outcome. These may be broadly categorized into challenges in coordinated action across agriculture and nutrition, in achievement of required improvements in agricultural production and food security, and in translating agricultural improvements into nutritional improvement.

A number of challenges to coordinated action across agriculture and nutrition are implicitly set out in the previous section. There are fundamental challenges in working effectively across traditionally separate disciplines and sectors which are enshrined in often competing government, research and other organizations, in different bodies of knowledge and world views, in different career and incentive structures, and in sectoral funding allocations [46, 47]. There are major challenges in getting policy and political commitment to bridge the two disciplines and sectors at all levels of work, from policy formulation and implementation to field operations. These challenges need to be specifically addressed as proposed by Fan et al. [42], with a search for clear 'win-win' opportunities across the divides (such as local sourcing for school feeding schemes) and with 'policy champions', 'civil society advocacy coalitions' and community and other decentralized efforts [46]. An underlying difficulty is the lack of sufficient good-quality research on agriculture-nutrition interactions and the lack of common metrics across the disciplinary and sectoral interfaces. Another core challenge is the achievement of greater gender empowerment – women play critical roles in agriculture and the integrated management of household resources for nutrition (as well as other goals).

Challenges in increasing agricultural production and improving food security have become increasingly apparent since the 2008 food spike, which results from a 'perfect storm' of interacting factors involving declining or stagnant productivity (as a result of low investment, increasing environmental pressures and increasing fossil fuel costs), increasing demand (from rising incomes and populations) and increasing instability (from environmental shocks, reduced stocks, and financial and physical speculation) [20, 48, 49]. Further rises in fuel prices, the negative effects of climate change on agriculture, and continuing population and dietary change with growing incomes pose further challenges to agricultural labor productivity and prices, particularly in poorer agrarian economies in the tropics – with both a general tightening of food availability and prices and increasing instability in both availability and market access. Unfortunately, these challenges strike at all three agriculture-nutrition pathways. Addressing them requires approaches that again cross disciplines and sectors in building resilience, diversity and nutritional effectiveness [50].

Finally, and drawing together the two previous sets of challenges, there are challenges in getting agricultural development to actually impact nutrition. These challenges arise for multiple reasons (and are well illustrated by the nutritional challenges in India) – for example the lack of gender empowerment in agricultural fora, challenges in getting changes in food security systems that impact the critical 1,000 days from conception, or limits to benefits from biofortification of staples where infants do not consume enough to get sufficient nutrient benefits even after biofortification, as well as the disciplinary and sectoral disconnects discussed earlier.

The challenges of improving agricultural-nutrition linkages to address the scandal of acute undernutrition are therefore very substantial. There is, however, considerable potential for gain with emerging new opportunities and, even with a marked lack of attention in the past, a strong record of achievement to build on. Increasing recognition of the importance of nutrition for human welfare and of the potential for nutritional measures to provide proxy measures for well-being is also likely to increase the importance of agriculture-nutrition linages in agricultural policies. There is much to play for.

Disclosure Statement

The author declares that no financial or other conflict of interest exists in relation to the content of the chapter.

References

1 United Nations: Road map towards the implementation of the United Nations Millennium Declaration. New York, United Nations, 2001.

2 United Nations: The Millennium Development Goals Report 2012. New York, United Nations, 2012.

3 Waage J, Banerji R, Campbell O, et al: The Millennium Development Goals: a cross-sectoral analysis and principles for goal setting after 2015. Lancet 2010;376:991–1023.

4 Headey D: Was the global food crisis really a crisis? Simulations versus self-reporting, IFPRI Discussion Paper 01087. Washington, International Food Policy Research Institute, 2011.

5 FAO, WFP, IFAD: The state of food insecurity in the world 2012. Economic growth is necessary but not sufficient to accelerate reduction of hunger and malnutrition. Rome, Food and Agriculture Organisation of the United Nations, 2012.

6 Committee on World Food Security: Global strategic framework for food security and nutrition: first version. Rome, Food and Agriculture Organisation of the United Nations, 2012.

7 Fan S, Brzeska J: The nexus between agriculture and nutrition: do growth patterns and conditional factors matter? 2020 Conference: Leveraging Agriculture for Improving Nutrition and Health; New Delhi, February 2011. Washington, International Food Policy Research Institute, 2011.

8 Hawkes C, Turner R, Waage J: Current and planned research on agriculture for improved nutrition: a mapping and a gap analysis, a report for DFID, LCIRAH. London, 2012.

9 Headey D: Turning economic growth into nutrition-sensitive growth, 2020 Conference: Leveraging Agriculture for Improving Nutrition and Health; New Delhi, February 2011. Washington, International Food Policy Research Institute, 2011.

10 Hoddinott J: Agriculture, health, and nutrition: toward conceptualizing the linkages; in Fan S, Pandya-Lorch R (eds): Reshaping Agriculture for Nutrition and Health. Washington, International Food Policy Research Institute, 2012, pp 13–20.

11 Pinstrup-Andersen P: The food system and its interaction with human health and nutrition; in Fan S, Pandya-Lorch R (eds): Reshaping Agriculture for Nutrition and Health. Washington, International Food Policy Research Institute, 2012, pp 21–29.

12 World Bank: From agriculture to nutrition: pathways, synergies and outcomes Washington, World Bank, 2007.

13 Dorward AR, Dangour AD: Agriculture and health. BMJ 2012;344:d7834.

14 Johnston BF, Mellor JW: The role of agriculture in economic development. Am Econ Rev 1961;51:566–593.

15 Mellor JW (ed): Agriculture on the Road to Industrialization. Baltimore, IFPRI/John Hopkins Press, 1995.

16 Timmer CP: The agricultural transformation; in Chenery H, Srinivasan TN (eds): The Handbook of Development Economics. Amsterdam, North Holland, 1988, vol 1, pp 275–331.

17 Christiaensen L, Demery L, Kuhl J: The (evolving) role of agriculture in poverty reduction – an empirical perspective. J Dev Econ 2011;96:239–254.

18 Dorward AR: Agricultural labour productivity, food prices and sustainable development impacts and indicators. Food Policy 2012;39: 40–50.

19 Collier P, Dercon S: African agriculture in 50 years: smallholders in a rapidly changing world? Expert Meeting on How to Feed the World in 2050, Food and Agriculture Organization of the United Nations, Economic and Social Development Department; Rome, June 2009.

20 Piesse J, Thirtle C: Three bubbles and a panic: an explanatory review of recent food commodity price events. Food Policy 2009;34: 119–129.

21 Dorward AR: Getting real about food prices. Dev Policy Rev 2011;29:647–664.

22 Webb P, Block S: Support for agriculture during economic transformation: impacts on poverty and undernutrition. Proc Natl Acad Sci 2012;109:12309–12314.

23 Ecker O, Breisinger C, Pauw K: Growth is good, but is not enough to improve nutrition, 2020 Conference: Leveraging Agriculture for Improving Nutrition and Health; New Delhi, February 2011. Washington, International Food Policy Research Institute, 2012, pp 47–54.

24 Pauw K, Thurlow J: The role of agricultural growth in reducing poverty and hunger: the case of Tanzania, 2020 Conference: Leveraging Agriculture for Improving Nutrition and Health; New Delhi, February 2011. Washington, International Food Policy Research Institute, 2012, pp 55–63.

25 Evenson R, Gollin D: The Green Revolution: an end of century perspective. Science 2003; 300:758–762.

26 Food and Agriculture Organisation of the United Nations: The state of food insecurity in the world: how does international price volatility affect domestic economies and food security? Rome, Food and Agriculture Organisation of the United Nations, 2011.

27 Ivanic M, Martin W: Implications of higher global food prices for poverty in low-income countries. Agric Econ 2008;39:405–416.

28 Brinkman H-J, de Pee S, Sanogo I, et al: High food prices and the global financial crisis have reduced access to nutritious food and worsened nutritional status and health. J Nutr 2010;140:153S–161S.

29 Dorward AR: The short and medium term impacts of rises in staple food prices. Food Security 2012;4:633–645.

30 Compton J, Wiggins S, Keats S: Impact of the global food crisis on the poor: what is the evidence? London, Overseas Development Institute, 2010.

31 Block S, Kiess L, Webb P, et al: Macro shocks and micro outcomes: child nutrition during Indonesia's crisis. Econ Hum Biol 2004;2: 21–44.

32 Torlesse H, Kiess L, Bloem MW: Association of household rice expenditure with child nutritional status indicates a role for macroeconomic food policy in combating malnutrition. J Nutr 2003;133:1320–1325.

33 Westby A, Coote C, Tomlins K: Increasing the production, availability, and consumption of vitamin A-rich sweet potato in Mozambique and Uganda, cited by Hawkes and Ruel. Natural Resources Institute, University of Greenwich, Greenwich, 2011.

34 Hawkes C, Ruel MT: Value chains for nutrition, in Fan S, Pandya-Lorch R (eds): Reshaping Agriculture for Nutrition and Health. Washington, International Food Policy Research Institute, 2012, pp 73–81.

35 Girard AW, Self JL, McAuliffe C, Olude O: The effects of household food production strategies on the health and nutrition outcomes of women and young children: a systematic review. Paediatr Perinat Epidemiol 2012;26(suppl 1):205–222.

36 Masset E, Haddad L, Cornelius A, Isaza-Castro J: Effectiveness of agricultural interventions that aim to improve nutritional status of children: systematic review. BMJ 2012;344:d8222.

37 Berti PR, Krasevec J, FitzGerald S: A review of the effectiveness of agriculture interventions in improving nutrition outcomes. Public Health Nutr 2004;7:599–609.

38 Ward M, Santos P: Looking beyond the plot: the nutritional impact of fertilizer policy; in Agric Appl Econ Assoc 2010 AAEA, CAES & WAEA Joint Ann Meet, Denver, July 2010.

39 Dorward AR, Kydd J, Morrison J, Urey I: A policy agenda for pro-poor agricultural growth. World Dev 2004;32:73–89.

40 Paarlberg R: Governing the dietary transition: linking agriculture, nutrition, and health, 2020 Conference: Leveraging Agriculture for Improving Nutrition and Health; New Delhi, February 2011. Washington, International Food Policy Research Institute, 2011, pp 191–199.

41 Herforth A, Jones A, Pinstrup-Andersen P: Prioritizing nutrition in agriculture and rural development: guiding principles for operational investments; Health, Nutrition, and Population (HNP) Discussion Paper. Washington, World Bank, 2012.

42 Fan S, Pandya-Lorch R, Fritschel H: Leveraging agriculture for improving nutrition and health: the way forward, 2020 conference: Leveraging Agriculture for Improving Nutrition and Health; New Delhi, February 2011. Washington, International Food Policy Research Institute, 2011, pp 201–207.

43 Gong Y, Hounsa A, Egal S, et al: Postweaning exposure to aflatoxin results in impaired child growth: a longitudinal study in Benin, West Africa. Environ Health Perspect 2004; 112:1334–1338.

44 Williams JH, Phillips TD, Jolly PE, et al: Human aflatoxicosis in developing countries: a review of toxicology, exposure, potential health consequences, and interventions. Am J Clin Nutr 2004;80:1106–1122.

45 Khlangwiset P, Shephard GS, Wu F: Aflatoxins and growth impairment: a review. Crit Rev Toxicol 2011;41:740–755.

46 Benson T: Cross-sectoral coordination in the public sector: a challenge to leveraging agriculture for improving nutrition and health, 2020 Conference: Leveraging Agriculture for Improving Nutrition and Health; New Delhi, February 2011. Washington, International Food Policy Research Institute, 2011, pp 145–153.

47 von Braun J, Ruel MT, Gillespie S: Bridging the gap between the agriculture and health sectors, 2020 Conference: Leveraging Agriculture for Improving Nutrition and Health; New Delhi, February 2011. Washington, International Food Policy Research Institute, 2011, pp 183–189.

48 Godfray HCJ, Beddington JR, Crute IR, et al: Food security: the challenge of feeding 9 billion people. Science 2010;327:812–818.

49 Headey D, Fan S: Reflections on the global food crisis. How did it happen? How has it hurt? And how can we prevent the next one? Research monograph 165. Washington, International Food Policy Research Institute, 2010.

50 Naylor R: Expanding the boundaries of agricultural development. Food Security 2011;3: 233–251.

Evidence on Interventions and Field Experiences

Black RE, Singhal A, Uauy R (eds): International Nutrition: Achieving Millennium Goals and Beyond.
Nestlé Nutr Inst Workshop Ser, vol 78, pp 111–120, (DOI: 10.1159/000354949)
Nestec Ltd., Vevey/S. Karger AG., Basel, © 2014

Long-Term Consequences of Nutrition and Growth in Early Childhood and Possible Preventive Interventions

Linda S. Adair

Department of Nutrition, Gillings School of Global Public Health, University of North Carolina at Chapel Hill, Chapel Hill, NC, USA

Abstract

Maternal nutritional deficiencies and excesses during pregnancy, and faster infant weight gain in the first 2 years of life are associated with increased risk of noncommunicable diseases (NCDs) in adulthood. The first 1,000 days of life (from conception until the child reaches age 2 years) represent a vulnerable period for programming of NCD risk, and are an important target for prevention of adult disease. This paper takes a developmental perspective to identify periconception, pregnancy, and infancy nutritional stressors, and to discuss mechanisms through which they influence later disease risk with the goal of informing age-specific interventions. Low- and middle-income countries need to address the dual burden of under- and overnutrition by implementing interventions to promote growth and enhance survival and intellectual development without increasing chronic disease risk. In the absence of good evidence from long-term follow-up of early life interventions, current recommendations for early life prevention of adult disease presume that interventions designed to optimize pregnancy outcomes and promote healthy infant growth and development will also reduce chronic disease risk. These include an emphasis on optimizing maternal nutrition prior to pregnancy, micronutrient adequacy in the preconception period and during pregnancy, promotion of breastfeeding and high-quality complementary foods, and prevention of obesity in childhood and adolescence.

© 2014 Nestec Ltd., Vevey/S. Karger AG, Basel

Introduction

Adult health, intellectual capacity, and well-being have developmental origins beginning in the preconception period. Poor prenatal growth and development manifested as low birthweight (LBW) and small size for gestational age (SGA)

at birth are strongly related to increased likelihood of adult short stature, reduced cognitive capacity, and lower educational attainment [1, 2]. A large body of animal and epidemiologic evidence also demonstrates that obesity and many adult noncommunicable diseases (NCDs) have origins as early as the periconception period. In particular, inadequate fetal nutrition, usually related to poor maternal nutritional status or impaired placental transport, is a key early life exposure that can elicit anatomical, hormonal, and physiological changes to enhance short-term survival but contribute to NCDs when nutritional resources are more plentiful later in life [2]. At the other end of the nutrition spectrum, maternal obesity, excess pregnancy weight gain and an oversupply of nutrients to the fetus relate to higher offspring birthweight, increased adiposity, and alterations in glucose metabolism in the offspring which in turn, increase risk of cardiometabolic disease risk later in life [3]. After birth, the trajectory of growth influences adult body size and composition, cognitive and brain function, and cardiometabolic and other NCD risk [2].

Given the importance of early development for adult health, it is vital to identify age-specific interventions that not only improve health but also optimize long-term health and human capital. Taking a life cycle perspective, the main goal of this chapter is to briefly synthesize information about major stressors, mechanisms through which they program disease risk, specific consequences, implications for intervention, and quality of the evidence base to support interventions, with a focus on the vulnerable periods that characterize the first 1,000 days of life. Owing to the extensive literature in these areas, recent reviews are cited to link readers to original sources. Optimizing early life nutrition is critical for attaining the Millennium Development Goals (MDGs), but it takes on an additional importance given the rapidity of economic development and the spread of obesity and NCDs worldwide.

Periconception

Maternal nutritional status at conception influences offspring health and development because the mother creates the earliest environmental exposures for the developing individual. Maternal short stature and low body mass index (BMI) are associated with increased risk of intrauterine growth restriction (IUGR) and LBW in the offspring [4]. Prepregnancy obesity is related to higher fetal growth rates, higher adiposity, and larger size for gestational age at birth [3]. Periconception maternal micronutrient status influences placental development, development of fetal tissue, and regulatory processes [5, 6]. Maternal weight status at conception can alter expression of genes implicated in the regulation of growth (insulin-like growth factors), and circulating levels of micronutrients, especially methyl donors, may influence DNA methylation in the early embryo to set the course of fetal development [7].

Since maternal nutrition at conception is important, some prevention efforts must focus on optimizing prepregnancy maternal nutritional status. This requires an intergenerational focus as well as attention to current conditions, because maternal stature, body composition, and response to dietary intake are influenced by her own early development. Delaying first birth and lengthening pregnancy intervals may also improve nutritional status at conception and reduce risk of IUGR [8, 9]. Recent initiatives, including the Bill and Melinda Gates Foundation's 'Start with a Girl: A New Agenda for Global Health' and the Center for Global Development's 'Girls Count: A Global Investment and Action Agenda' have focused on young girls as an important target for improving long-term offspring health. This emphasis is also important in light of the sharp increases in obesity in postmenarcheal girls in several low- and middle-income countries, such as South Africa and Guatemala [10], putting young women at risk for pregnancies complicated by obesity as well as micronutrient deficiencies.

The focus on maternal micronutrient status can be more immediate. Since micronutrient status is largely influenced by current diet, adolescent girls and young women can be targeted for prepregnancy interventions that may include nutrition education, or food-based or micronutrient supplements. Given current understanding of mechanisms, multiple micronutrients are important for many health outcomes, but methyl donors are critical not only for their role in reducing neural tube defects, but also for their epigenetic effects [5].

The relationship of periconceptional nutrition (up to 12 weeks' gestation) to birth outcomes and the effectiveness of short-term interventions targeted to that period were recently reviewed [6]. While the authors found evidence of significant associations of poor maternal nutrition status (low BMI, low iodine intake, iron deficiency anemia) with risk of IUGR or LBW, they also concluded that evidence supporting a link between maternal periconception interventions and infant birth outcomes was of low quality and inconsistent except for reduction of neural tube defects by folate.

Pregnancy

An extensive literature documents how maternal weight status, gestational weight gain, and micronutrient status relate to birth outcomes [5]. Fetal nutritional stressors include inadequate or excess energy and specific nutrients to supply building blocks for developing organs or regulate development and metabolic processes. Nutrient supply reflects maternal stores, dietary intake and placental function. Maternal short stature, underweight and inadequate pregnancy weight gain are related to lower birthweight and smaller size for gestational age, while maternal overweight and obesity (independent of, and with gestational diabetes) are related to greater newborn adiposity and larger size for gestational age [3].

Limited or excess energy and nutrients can influence fetal growth and long-term health and susceptibility to disease through several pathways. Nutrient restriction may differentially limit organ and tissue growth. For example, protein restriction produces relatively larger deficits in skeletal muscle and kidneys than in heart or brain [2]. Such deficits have long-term consequences because they are difficult to reverse later in life, and smaller organs (e.g. kidneys with fewer nephrons or a pancreas with fewer β-cells) may have reduced functional capacity [11]. Yajnik et al. [12] have noted the phenomenon of the 'thin-fat' India baby who, following maternal undernutrition, is born with large deficits in skeletal muscle but not adiposity. These babies are at increased risk of later developing insulin resistance and diabetes, emphasizing the importance of fetal body composition [13].

An inadequate supply of nutrients may trigger a cascade of metabolic adaptations that enhance survival in the short run but increase risk of metabolic diseases when nutrients are no longer in short supply. According to the 'thrifty phenotype hypothesis' [14, 15], glucocorticoid exposure subsequent to maternal stress or poor nutritional status may program the insulin and hypothalamic-pituitary-adrenal (HPA) axes for high levels of metabolic efficiency [2], leading to impaired glucose metabolism and insulin resistance in the face of dietary excesses later in life. Gestational diabetes creates an intrauterine environment with high levels of glucose and insulin, resulting in fetal macrosomia and altered fetal and newborn glucose regulation. Growing evidence suggests that maternal obesity, even without gestational diabetes, is a risk factor for child obesity through a pathway related to fetal overnutrition [3].

Specific nutrients may alter gene expression in regulatory pathways related to the HPA axis, glucose metabolism, blood pressure and fetal growth, with important consequences for NCDs later in life. Experimental animal studies show specific effects of maternal intake of methyl donors with implications for the development of adiposity [7], but evidence from human studies is quite limited [16]. Dutch adults prenatally exposed to famine had altered patterns of DNA methylation [17], and increased IGF gene methylation was observed in blood from 17-month-old children whose mothers had taken periconception folic acid [18], but these studies are unable to isolate effects of prenatal exposures. Studies of newborns show inconsistent associations of maternal diet with methylation in cord blood: maternal folate intake was not related, but choline intake was related to cord blood methylation in a folate-replete population in the US [19]. A recent pilot study in the Gambia found that micronutrient supplementation reduced methylation levels at 2 imprinted growth-related loci [20], but evidence from other trials is lacking. A concern about folate supplementation was raised based on the Pune, India, study [21], where high maternal folate and low vitamin B_{12} during pregnancy were associated with increased adiposity and insulin resistance in the offspring, but a Nepal study found no effect of maternal folate or other micronutrient supplements on insulin resistance in school-aged offspring [22]. Another relevant consideration is that since epigenetic marks are preserved across generations, exposures in pregnant women may affect not only their sons and daughters but also their grandchildren [7].

A recent collection of systematic reviews and meta-analyses evaluated the effects of a wide range of maternal interventions on birth outcomes [23]. In most cases, the evidence base for effects was evaluated as weak and inconsistent, but numerous studies showed modest effects of maternal iron, calcium, vitamin D, vitamin B_6, n-3 long-chain polyunsaturated fatty acids, multiple micronutrient, and balanced protein-energy supplementation supplements on birthweight (50–100 g) and/or reduction of LBW (15–20%).

Based on strong evidence linking birthweight to adult size, body composition, and NCD risk, we would expect such improvements in birthweight to have important, but modest long-term benefits related to NCDs. For example, in a pooled analysis from 5 low- and middle-income countries, 1 kg higher birthweight was related (after adjustment for adult size) to 1.8 mm Hg lower systolic blood pressure and about 0.6 mmol/l lower blood glucose [24]. However, it is notable that each kg of birthweight related to 3.3 cm of adult height, 0.3 years of attained schooling and 208 g of birthweight in the next generation, stressing the importance of prenatal growth for these aspects of health and well-being.

The implications of interventions benefitting birthweight are also limited because birthweight fails to tell the full story of early life risk development. In addition to organ-specific deficits that may not be reflected in birthweight, alterations in metabolism and long-term disease risk occur in the absence of significant effects on birthweight [25]. Understanding the consequences of such alterations will require more nuanced assessments of infant nutritional status of birth, particularly since altered fetal metabolism may act through altered susceptibility to later environmental influences.

In sum, prevention prior to and during pregnancy needs to focus on maternal health, starting with the prior generation to promote good linear growth and optimal body composition, and then on ensuring adequate nutrient stores, adequate macro- and micronutrient intakes to meet maternal and fetal needs, adequate pregnancy weight gain, and freedom from stress and infections.

Infancy

The well-established associations of infant underweight and stunting with adult stature, school attainment and productivity [26] have provided a strong rationale for many interventions aimed at improving early child growth. A goal of many postnatal interventions is to enhance weight gain among children born SGA-age or to promote recovery from severe or moderate malnutrition because compensatory growth is associated with reduced morbidity and mortality, and improved cognitive development [27, 28]. However, 'rapid growth' during infancy is sometimes associated with increased risk of obesity, insulin resistance, and elevated blood pressure in childhood and adulthood [29]. A key concern is thus whether benefits of interventions which promote faster growth in low- and middle-income countries outweigh the possible long-term risks. Critical questions relate to age when rapid weight gain occurs and whether weight gain is accompanied by linear growth and accumulation of lean mass as well as fat tissue.

Studies of birth cohorts in five low- and-middle income countries (Brazil, Guatemala, India, The Philippines and South Africa) explored these questions in relation to adult stature, body composition, school attainment, blood pressure and plasma glucose. Initial findings were that higher weight-for-age z score at 2 years is related to taller adult stature, higher attained schooling, higher BMI, but lower blood pressure and blood glucose [30]. In subsequent work, the COHORTS team disentangled the consequences of faster linear growth versus relative weight gain at different ages [31]. Faster linear growth through early childhood was more strongly related to taller young adult stature and better attained schooling, but only weakly related to higher BP, and unrelated to fasting glucose. Faster relative weight gain was related to higher adult BMI, fat and fat-free mass, blood pressure and fasting glucose. The associations with adverse outcomes were weak in the first 2 years but strengthened with age: relative weight gain after mid-childhood was a much more important risk factor for later chronic disease risk than was relative weight gain in the first 2 years. Of particular note is the beneficial effect of early weight gain on the development of fat-free mass, emphasizing the importance of body composition rather than weight gain alone. The study also underscores the importance of early linear growth.

It is assumed that promoting healthy postnatal growth will also promote long-term health. Key factors are optimal diet, responsive care, and protection from infection [32]. For the young infant, this means breastfeeding according to well-established guidelines. An extensive literature documents the benefits of breastfeeding for promoting growth, and reducing morbidity and mortality. The long-term effects of breastfeeding are more controversial, and causal inferences are limited by lack of randomized controlled trials. Some studies relate breastfeeding to lower risk of obesity and NCDs, while other studies show no effects [33], but no studies show any adverse effects.

Highly effective strategies to improve child growth have yet to be developed. Bhutta et al. [32] concluded that food supplements in food-insecure populations increase height-for-age z scores, but recent Cochrane reviews concluded that community-based supplementary feeding had only small or negligible effects on growth of children under 5 years of age [34], and home fortification of foods with micronutrient powders improved iron status but did not influence growth [35]. Zinc supplementation appears to be one of the more effective means to improve linear growth [36].

Composition and quality of the weaning diet may also be important. The WHO recently convened a panel to examine effects of complementary feeding on development of NCDs [37]. Reviews of specific aspects of diet with potential long-term health consequences suggest roles for excess protein intake in the development of obesity, excess sodium intake in the development of hypertension, and high intake or dietary imbalances of fat composition for atherogenic lipid profiles, but most studies cited a lack of clear evidence from follow-up of controlled trials.

Few studies have directly evaluated the effects of childhood nutrition interventions on later risk of NCDs [38]. In Guatemala, adults who were exposed to a protein and multiple micronutrient-fortified food supplement (atole) had lower fasting glucose and systolic blood pressure when exposed to atole from 24–60 months, higher HDL cholesterol and lower triglycerides when exposed during gestation and the first 3 years. Atole was unrelated to adult total or LDL cholesterol [39]. In the Gambia, follow-up of a protein-energy supplement trial in the second half of pregnancy at ages 11–17 years showed marginally lower fasting glucose but no differences in blood pressure, body composition or cholesterol levels in those exposed to supplements [40]. In a shorter-term follow-up of the Maternal and Infant Nutrition Interventions trial in Bangladesh, multiple micronutrient supplements provided to rural women during pregnancy did not affect offspring body composition at 54 months of age [41].

Discussion and Conclusions

MDG 1 focuses on the reduction of hunger, which remains unacceptably high in Sub-Saharan Africa and Southern Asia outside of India and is increasing in southern Africa. Large urban-rural and wealth-related disparities in underweight prevalence remain [42]. At the same time, rates of obesity and chronic disease are rising rapidly in low- and middle-income countries with the most dramatic increases among the poor [43]. Thus, while the primary focus for attaining MDGs needs to remain on reducing mortality and undernutrition, the MDG call for more emphasis on nutrition in the development agenda could also benefit from a stronger focus on linear growth and a forward look to the prevention of adult disease.

Prevention of IUGR and stunting may not be sufficient since long-term disease risk varies across the full spectrum of early life nutrition. Optimal diet composition for prevention of early obesity is also important, although the evidence base for this needs development as research is needed to define an optimal weaning and early child diet that promotes linear growth and lean body mass while minimizing excess adiposity.

By identifying vulnerable periods and tailoring prevention efforts to those vulnerabilities, we can try to capitalize on the same developmental plasticity that alters susceptibility to disease [44]. We know what the vulnerabilities are, and we know quite a bit about how they influence NCDs in the long run. Our knowledge gap reflects inadequate information on effective interventions. In the absence of a strong evidence base on how early life interventions relate to adult outcomes (particularly NCDs), at present we must presume that interventions aimed at improving maternal, fetal, and infant growth will also be effective for improving adult outcomes. The limitations in effective strategies for short-term maternal and child health are thus shared when considering long-term effects.

Disclosure Statement

The author declares that no financial or other conflict of interest exists in relation to the content of the chapter.

References

1 Victora CG, Adair L, Fall C, et al: Maternal and child undernutrition: consequences for adult health and human capital. Lancet 2008; 371:340–357.
2 Gluckman P, Hanson M (eds): Developmental Origins of Health and Disease. Cambridge, Cambridge University Press, 2006.
3 Fall C: Maternal nutrition: effects on health in the next generation. Indian J Med Res 2009;130:593–599.
4 Kramer MS: Determinants of low birth weight: methodological assessment and meta-analysis. Bull World Health Organ 1987;65: 663–737.
5 Wu G, Imhoff-Kunsch B, Girard AW: Biological mechanisms for nutritional regulation of maternal health and fetal development. Paediatr Perinat Epidemiol 2012;26(suppl 1): 4–26.
6 Ramakrishnan U, Grant F, Goldenberg T, et al: Effect of women's nutrition before and during early pregnancy on maternal and infant outcomes: a systematic review. Paediatr Perinat Epidemiol 2012;26(suppl 1):285–301.
7 Hochberg Z, Feil R, Constancia M, et al: Child health, developmental plasticity, and epigenetic programming. Endocr Rev 2010; 32:159–224.

8   Gibbs CM, Wendt A, Peters S, et al: The im-
    pact of early age at first childbirth on mater-
    nal and infant health. Paediatr Perinat Epide-
    miol 2012;26(suppl 1):259–284.

9   Wendt A, Gibbs CM, Peters S, et al: Impact
    of increasing inter-pregnancy interval on ma-
    ternal and infant health. Paediatr Perinat Epi-
    demiol 2012;26(suppl 1):239–258.

10 Kimani-Murage EW, Kahn K, Pettifor JM, et
    al: Predictors of adolescent weight status and
    central obesity in rural South Africa. Public
    Health Nutr 2011;14:1114–1122.

11 Barker DJ, Bagby SP, Hanson MA: Mecha-
    nisms of disease: in utero programming in
    the pathogenesis of hypertension. Nat Clin
    Pract Nephrol 2006;2:700–707.

12 Yajnik CS, Fall CH, Coyaji KJ, et al: Neonatal
    anthropometry: the thin-fat Indian baby. The
    Pune Maternal Nutrition Study. Int J Obes
    Relat Metab Disord 2003;27:173–180.

13 Joglekar CV, Fall CH, Deshpande VU, et al:
    Newborn size, infant and childhood growth,
    and body composition and cardiovascular
    disease risk factors at the age of 6 years: the
    Pune Maternal Nutrition Study. Int J Obes
    (Lond) 2007;31:1534–1544.

14 Prentice AM: Early influences on human en-
    ergy regulation: thrifty genotypes and thrifty
    phenotypes. Physiol Behav 2005;86:640–645.

15 Wells JC: The thrifty phenotype: an adapta-
    tion in growth or metabolism? Am J Hum
    Biol 2010;23:65–75.

16 Dominguez-Salas P, Cox SE, Prentice AM, et
    al: Maternal nutritional status, C(1) metabo-
    lism and offspring DNA methylation: a re-
    view of current evidence in human subjects.
    Proc Nutr Soc 2012;71:154–165.

17 Tobi EW, Slagboom PE, van Dongen J, et al:
    Prenatal famine and genetic variation are in-
    dependently and additively associated with
    DNA methylation at regulatory loci within
    IGF2/H19. PLoS One 2012;7:e37933.

18 Steegers-Theunissen RP, Obermann-Borst
    SA, Kremer D, et al: Periconceptional mater-
    nal folic acid use of 400 microg per day is re-
    lated to increased methylation of the IGF2
    gene in the very young child. PLoS One 2009;
    4:e7845.

19 Boeke CE, Baccarelli A, Kleinman KP, et al:
    Gestational intake of methyl donors and
    global LINE-1 DNA methylation in maternal
    and cord blood: prospective results from a
    folate-replete population. Epigenetics 2012;7:
    253–260.

20 Cooper WN, Khulan B, Owens S, et al: DNA
    methylation profiling at imprinted loci after
    periconceptional micronutrient supplemen-
    tation in humans: results of a pilot random-
    ized controlled trial. FASEB J 2012;26:1782–
    1790.

21 Yajnik CS, Deshpande SS, Jackson AA, et al:
    Vitamin B12 and folate concentrations dur-
    ing pregnancy and insulin resistance in the
    offspring: the Pune Maternal Nutrition
    Study. Diabetologia 2008;51:29–38.

22 Stewart CP, Christian P, Schulze KJ, et al:
    Low maternal vitamin B-12 status is associ-
    ated with offspring insulin resistance regard-
    less of antenatal micronutrient supplementa-
    tion in rural Nepal. J Nutr 2011;141:
    1912–1917.

23 Special Issue: Improving maternal, newborn,
    and child health outcomes through better
    designed policies and programs that enhance
    the nutrition of women. Paediatr Perinat Epi-
    demiol 2012;26:1–325.

24 Martorell R, Horta BL, Adair LS, et al:
    Weight gain in the first two years of life is an
    important predictor of schooling outcomes in
    pooled analyses from five birth cohorts from
    low- and middle-income countries. J Nutr
    2010;140:348–354.

25 Li C, Schlabritz-Loutsevitch NE, Hubbard
    GB, et al: Effects of maternal global nutrient
    restriction on fetal baboon hepatic insulin-
    like growth factor system genes and gene
    products. Endocrinology 2009;150:4634–
    4642.

26 Dewey KG, Begum K: Long-term conse-
    quences of stunting in early life. Matern
    Child Nutr 2011;7(suppl 3):5–18.

27 Victora CG, Barros FC, Horta BL, et al:
    Short-term benefits of catch-up growth for
    small-for-gestational-age infants. Int J Epide-
    miol 2001;30:1325–1330.

28 Walker SP, Wachs TD, Gardner JM, et al:
    Child development: risk factors for adverse
    outcomes in developing countries. Lancet
    2007;369:145–157.

29 Ong KK, Loos RJ: Rapid infancy weight gain
    and subsequent obesity: systematic reviews
    and hopeful suggestions. Acta Paediatr 2006;
    95:904–908.

30 Victora CG, Adair L, Fall C, et al: Maternal
    and child undernutrition: consequences for
    adult health and human capital. Lancet 2008;
    371:340–357.

31 Adair L, Fall C, Osmond C, et al: Associations of linear growth and relative weight gain during early life with adult health and human capital in countries of low and middle income: findings from five birth cohort studies. Lancet 2013;382:525–534.

32 Bhutta ZA, Ahmed T, Black RE, et al: What works? Interventions for maternal and child undernutrition and survival. Lancet 2008; 371:417–440.

33 Horta B, Bahl R, Martinés J, et al: Evidence on the long-term effects of breastfeeding: systematic reviews and meta-analysis. Geneva, World Health Organization, 2007.

34 Sguassero Y, de Onis M, Bonotti AM, Carroli G: Community-based supplementary feeding for promoting the growth of children under five years of age in low and middle income countries. Cochrane Database Syst Rev 2012;CD005039.

35 De-Regil LM, Suchdev PS, Vist GE, et al: Home fortification of foods with multiple micronutrient powders for health and nutrition in children under two years of age. Cochrane Database Syst Rev 2011;CD008959.

36 Imdad A, Bhutta ZA: Effect of preventive zinc supplementation on linear growth in children under 5 years of age in developing countries: a meta-analysis of studies for input to the lives saved tool. BMC Public Health 2011;11(suppl 3):S22.

37 Focus on Complementary Feeding and Dietary Prevention of Non-Communicable Diseases – Reports from the WHO/Regione Puglia Workshop. Nutr Metab Cardiovasc Dis 2012;22:763–928.

38 Hawkesworth S: Conference on 'Multidisciplinary approaches to nutritional problems'. Postgraduate Symposium. Exploiting dietary supplementation trials to assess the impact of the prenatal environment on CVD risk. Proc Nutr Soc 2009;68:78–88.

39 Stein AD, Wang M, Ramirez-Zea M, et al: Exposure to a nutrition supplementation intervention in early childhood and risk factors for cardiovascular disease in adulthood: evidence from Guatemala. Am J Epidemiol 2006;164:1160–1170.

40 Hawkesworth S, Walker CG, Sawo Y, et al: Nutritional supplementation during pregnancy and offspring cardiovascular disease risk in The Gambia. Am J Clin Nutr 2011;94: 1853S–1860S.

41 Khan AI, Kabir I, Hawkesworth S, et al: Early invitation to food and/or multiple micronutrient supplementation in pregnancy does not affect body composition in offspring at 54 months: follow-up of the MINIMat randomised trial, Bangladesh. Matern Child Nutr, E-pub ahead of print.

42 UNICEF: The Millennium Development Goals Report 20122102. New York, United Nations, 2012.

43 Popkin BM, Adair LS, Ng SW: Global nutrition transition and the pandemic of obesity in developing countries. Nutr Rev 2012;70: 3–21.

44 Gluckman PD, Hanson MA, Low FM: The role of developmental plasticity and epigenetics in human health. Birth Defects Res C Embryo Today 2011;93:12–18.

Evidence on Interventions and Field Experiences

Black RE, Singhal A, Uauy R (eds): International Nutrition: Achieving Millennium Goals and Beyond.
Nestlé Nutr Inst Workshop Ser, vol 78, pp 121–122, (DOI: 10.1159/000354950)
Nestec Ltd., Vevey/S. Karger AG., Basel, © 2014

Summary on Evidence on Interventions and Field Experiences

The second session of the workshop focused on the evidence to support interventions and programs that will help achieve the MDGs and other health benefits. *Zulfiqar Bhutta* presented a comprehensive review of potential interventions for women and children. Among the maternal interventions, iron supplementation in pregnancy was found to reduce anemia and low birthweight, but supplementation with a broader set of micronutrients has a greater effect, compared with iron and folic acid, on birthweight and the proportion of babies born small for gestational age (SGA). Provision of balanced protein-energy supplements in pregnancy for undernourished women also reduces the incidence of SGA. Among the interventions for children, counseling and support of mothers has resulted in substantial increases in exclusive breastfeeding in the first 6 months of life and in continued breastfeeding thereafter and in improved complementary feeding. Vitamin A and zinc supplements have been shown to reduce infectious disease morbidity and mortality in children. *Usha Ramakrishnan* provided additional evidence on maternal interventions. Antenatal calcium supplementation in calcium-deficient women in pregnancy reduces the risk of eclampsia, the second most important cause of maternal deaths, and reduces preterm births, the second leading cause of child deaths. She also indicated that her review found that antenatal zinc or omega-3 fatty acids reduced the risk of preterm birth. *Parul Christian* presented her analyses on the consequences of fetal growth restriction (indicated by being born SGA). Compared to births that were appropriate size for their gestational age, babies who were SGA and full term had twice the risk of being stunted later in childhood; babies who were SGA and preterm had five times the risk of stunting. She reaffirmed the role of balanced protein-energy supplementation, iron and multiple micronutrients in pregnancy to prevent SGA, as mentioned by *Zulfiqar Bhutta* and *Usha Ramak-*

rishnan, and its consequences for stunting. *Linda Adair* discussed the relationships of maternal nutritional deficits in pregnancy and the rates of weight gain in childhood with noncommunicable diseases in adulthood. Insufficient nutrients in pregnancy result in fetal adaptations that enhance survival in childhood but increase the risk of metabolic diseases later in life. Analyses by the COHORTS group have shown that faster weight gain relative to increase in height, especially in children after 2 years of age, was related to higher adult body mass index, fat and fat-free mass, blood pressure and fasting glucose concentration. Finally, in a change of pace *Andrew Dorward* discussed how agricultural interventions can contribute to human nutrition and achievement of the MDGs. The potential for impact on health and nutrition of three overlapping agricultural pathways (development, own production and market) was considered likely, but the evidence for their effects is limited. He indicated the need for more rigorous research in this area.

Robert E. Black

Black RE, Singhal A, Uauy R (eds): International Nutrition: Achieving Millennium Goals and Beyond.
Nestlé Nutr Inst Workshop Ser, vol 78, pp 123–132, (DOI: 10.1159/000354951)
Nestec Ltd., Vevey/S. Karger AG., Basel, © 2014

The Global Epidemic of Noncommunicable Disease: The Role of Early-Life Factors

Atul Singhal

The Childhood Nutrition Research Centre, Institute of Child Health, University College London, London, UK

Abstract

The rapid increase in prevalence of noncommunicable diseases (NCDs) is probably the most important global health problem of the 21st century. Already in every region except Africa, NCDs account for greater mortality than communicable, maternal, perinatal and nutritional conditions combined. Although modifiable lifestyle behaviors in adult life are the main risk factors, substantial evidence now suggests that factors in early life also have a major role in the development of NCDs. For instance, breastfeeding and a slower pattern of infant weight gain have been shown to reduce the risk of obesity, cardiovascular disease and diabetes in both low-income and high-income countries. The mechanisms involved are poorly understood, but include epigenetic changes and resetting of endocrine systems that affect energy metabolism and appetite. These early life factors may interact with and exacerbate the detrimental effects of a sedentary lifestyle and energy-dense diets later in life. As a consequence, the impact of early-life factors on long-term health may be particularly important in low- and middle-income countries, which face the fastest increases in urbanization and greatest changes to lifestyle. Strategies to optimize infant nutrition could therefore make a major contribution to stemming the current global epidemic of NCD.

Introduction

Although meeting the Millennium Development Goals and the prevention of undernutrition remains a major problem in many populations, the rapid increase in noncommunicable disease (NCD) has now become the highest priority for global public health. According to the WHO, in 2008 approximately 63% of all deaths (36 out of 57 million per year) were due to NCDs, comprising of cardiovascular disease (CVD), diabetes, cancers and chronic respiratory disease [1]. Of these, nearly 80% (29 million) occurred in low- or middle-income countries, with CVD, including diabetes, being the most common. In fact, contrary to popular belief, most deaths from CVD (80%) occur in low- or middle-income countries rather than in richer populations [1].

Whilst modifiable behavioral factors such as tobacco use, insufficient physical activity, the harmful use of alcohol, and unhealthy diets are the major risk factors, research over the last 10 years has highlighted the key role of early life factors in the development of NCD [1, 2]. Factors in utero, early postnatal life and throughout childhood have been shown to affect CVD by influencing the propensity to risk factors such as obesity, diabetes, hypertension and dyslipidemia: the so-called developmental origins of adult disease hypothesis. Many of these factors, such as infant and childhood nutrition, are modifiable, raising the possibility that interventions in early life could help stem the current global epidemic of NCD. The present review considers the role of these early life factors in the development of NCDs, focusing on the impact of infant nutrition on CVD in low- and middle-income countries. The review aims to highlight the experimental evidence where available, briefly summarize the mechanisms involved, and consider the implications for public health.

The Developmental Origins of Noncommunicable Disease

Historically, the concept that factors in early life such as nutrition can affect, or program, the development of NCDs emerged from animal work in the 1930s. McCay [3] showed that rats whose growth was stunted by restricting their food intake had a lower incidence of tumors, kidney disease, vascular calcification and chronic pneumonia and consequently a substantial 35% increase in lifespan. Subsequently, in the 1980s observational studies suggested an association between suboptimal fetal growth (as measured by low birthweight) and long-term risk of CVD – the 'fetal origins' of adult disease hypothesis [4]. These observations have been replicated many times including several studies from Sub-Saharan Africa linking lower birthweight with higher blood pressure in childhood [as reviewed in 2]. Of particular interest has been the association of birthweight with long-term body composition [5, 6]. In general, in both high- and low-income countries, body size in early life (birthweight and faster infant weight gain) is more strongly associated with greater fat-free mass than fat mass in adults, while there are some data linking low birthweight with greater visceral or central fat [6].

These epidemiological data, along with studies linking prenatal nutrition (e.g. famine during pregnancy, antenatal protein and energy intake, and maternal micronutrient supplementation) with later risk of obesity and CVD, suggest that nutrition during pregnancy is a modifiable risk factor for NCDs [5, 6]. However, there is little experimental evidence to support a *causal* link between prenatal nutrition and long-term CVD [7]. In one such study, supplementation of Nepalese mothers with fifteen micronutrients (compared to controls given only iron and folic acid) lowered systolic blood pressure in the offspring at 2–3 years of age [8]. However, this finding has yet to be replicated and, interestingly, there was no effect on diastolic blood pressure. The lack of randomized controlled trials (RCTs) is likely to be particularly important for associations between both birthweight and infant growth and later fat-free mass. Indeed, it is not surprising that 'larger' individuals (in height, body frame and hence in fat-free mass) are both larger at birth and have faster rates of infant weight gain, since both exposure and outcome will be strongly influenced by the same genetic factors. Therefore, although there is substantial ongoing research in this this area, currently there is little experimental evidence to suggest that modifying prenatal factors such as nutrition can help prevent later NCD.

Early Postnatal Factors and the Prevention of Noncommunicable Disease

Evidence that early postnatal factors program later health was first obtained in 1970 when faster weight gain in the first 6 months after birth was found to be associated with obesity at age 6–8 years [as reviewed in 9]. More recently, follow-up of adolescents born prematurely and randomly assigned to formula or human milk provided the first experimental evidence to show that breast milk feeding had long-term benefits for CVD risk factors such as obesity, dyslipidemia, raised blood pressure, and insulin resistance [10, 11]. Subsequently, five meta-analyses have confirmed that breastfeeding is associated with approximately 20% lower risk of obesity [summarized in 12–15], an effect size which is comparable to interventions for obesity later in life [13] and which is likely to be important for populations rather than for individual health. Compared to those formula fed, breastfed infants had lower fat mass rather than fat-free mass, a difference evident from as early as the first year of life [14].

Data to support benefits of breastfeeding for CVD risk factors other than obesity are more limited. All four systematic reviews and meta-analyses on the long-term effects of breastfeeding published since 2005 (Dutch State Institute for Nutrition and Health 2005; WHO 2007; US Agency for Healthcare Research and Quality 2007, and the UK Scientific Advisory Committee on Nutrition

2011) [as summarized in 13] support a protective effect of breastfeeding against the risk of obesity but only the latter three suggested that breastfeeding reduced later blood pressure and risk of type 2 diabetes. However, all reviews highlighted the possibility of residual confounding in the studies included.

The issue of confounding has been considered in research from Brazil, where, unlike developed countries, breastfeeding is not associated with socioeconomic status [16]. Here, breastfeeding was associated with later IQ but not with blood pressure or BMI [16]. One explanation is that breastfeeding is only protective against obesity in the highest part of the BMI distribution [12], and such high levels of obesity are likely to be more common in the 'obesogenic' environment found in richer countries. Therefore, early-life factors may have a priming effect (for example by affecting appetite regulation – see below) but depend on an interaction with subsequent environment (e.g. an energy-dense diet) to produce effects on health. This potential interaction of early-life factors with later environment is supported by animal models which showed that adverse effects of maternal protein restriction and faster postnatal growth on obesity and lifespan were most marked in mice fed a high calorie, 'cafeteria' diet, after weaning rather than normal chow [17].

The issue of residual confounding in studies of breastfeeding was also addressed in a large-scale cluster-randomized trial in Belarus (the PROBIT study) [18]. This trial compared an intervention which promoted breastfeeding with a control group that received normal health care and found a lower risk of gastrointestinal infection and eczema in the intervention arm. At 6.5 years of age, IQ was higher in the intervention group, but there were no differences between randomized groups in blood pressure or fat mass [18]. However, it is important to note that because the intervention was designed to increase the degree and duration of exclusive breastfeeding and not its initiation, the study may be underpowered to detect differences in outcomes between breastfed and formula-fed infants [18]. Overall therefore, other than in infants born preterm, the evidence that breastfeeding has long-term benefits for CVD risk is almost entirely observational, a situation which, given the impossibility of RCTs directly comparing breastfeeding with formula feeding, is unlikely to change in the future.

The Role of Infant Growth in Programming Cardiovascular Disease

Various mechanisms have been proposed for the programming effects of breastfeeding including confounding by health behaviors that affect CVD risk, effects on appetite regulation, and the possibility of biologically active factors in human milk which could affect energy intake and metabolism [19]. However, perhaps the most extensively studied hypothesis is that the long-term cardiovascular benefits of breastfeeding are a consequence of slower growth and relative undernutrition in breastfed compared to formula-fed infants – the growth acceleration hypothesis [11].

Over the last decade, substantial evidence has accumulated from both animal and human studies to support the growth acceleration concept [9, 11]. These data include several studies from low- and middle-income countries such as the Seychelles, Brazil and South Africa [as reviewed in 20]. In India, for example, men and women living in New Delhi who had features of the metabolic syndrome (increased waist circumference, higher blood pressure, insulin resistance and dyslipidemia) had more rapid weight gain in infancy than controls [21]. However, the size of these programming effects in cohorts from low- and middle-income countries appears to be small with, for example, a 1-SD change in early growth predicting less than a 1% change in adult body fat [6]. In contrast, in a contemporary Western environment, approximately 20% of the population risk of overweight in childhood can be attributed being in the highest quintile for weight gain in infancy [as reviewed in 9]. Nonetheless, given the potential interaction of programming effects with later environment, and global changes in habitual diet and lifestyle, the contribution of infant growth to long-term health is likely to become increasingly important even in low-income countries.

Unlike potential programming effects of antenatal nutrition or breastfeeding, the hypothesis that *infant growth* affects long-term health is strongly supported by evidence from randomized, double-blind, clinical trials that can establish a causal link between exposure and outcome. For instance, adolescents born preterm and randomly assigned to a nutrient-enriched (preterm) formula that promoted infant growth had greater blood pressure and insulin and cholesterol concentrations than those assigned to less nutrient-dense diets (term formula or breast milk) [10, 11]. Similarly, compared to controls, infants born at term, but small for gestation, who were randomly assigned to nutrient-enriched formula for 6–8 months had higher blood pressure in childhood [22], and in two trials, greater body fat up to 8 years later [23]. Programming effects of infant growth are also seen in experimental studies in term infants with normal birthweight. In the European Childhood Obesity Study, a large, multicenter RCT, infants randomized to formulas with a higher protein concentration for the first year (which promoted faster weight and length gain) had greater BMI at 2 years of age than controls. Based on existing data from observational studies, the authors predicted that this would lead to a 13% increase in later risk of obesity [24]. Finally, in a trial from Chile, healthy full-term infants of mothers who had a BMI of >25, randomly assigned to a lower-protein formula from 3 to 12 months (1.65 g/100 kcal, 628 kcal/l) had lower BMI at age 2 years than those given a control formula (2.63 g/100 kcal, 656 kcal/l) [Inostroza et al., unpubl.]. The latter study clearly illustrates that infant growth/nutrition has programming effects on the risk of obesity in middle-income countries.

Complementary Feeding

Whether the timing and quality of complementary feeding has an impact on long-term health is more controversial than effects of infant growth. A recent systematic review suggested that earlier introduction of solids, and especially before 4 months, was associated with a greater risk of obesity especially in infants fed formula [15]. This observation is consistent with the hypothesis that breast-feeding has a priming effect, possibly by favorably affecting appetite regulation. Infants given formula in the first few months after birth would be more susceptible to overfeeding if given solids earlier, which in itself could lead to faster infant weight gain and hence greater susceptibility to long-term obesity. Alternatively, since these studies are all observational, there is a high possibility of confounding. For example, fussy eaters or infants genetically susceptible to have a higher appetite are both more likely to be given solids earlier and are at greater risk of later obesity. The lack of experimental data therefore considerably limits our understanding of the impact of complementary feeding on long-term health.

Growth in Childhood and Programming of Cardiovascular Disease

A similar lack of RCTs limits interpretation of evidence linking faster weight gain *in childhood* with later CVD. This finding has been seen in both high-income and low-income countries. For instance, faster weight gain in children older than 2 years was associated with increased risk of death from CVD in a cohort from Helsinki [as reviewed in 9], while follow-up of children in Delhi found that glucose intolerance and type 2 diabetes were more common in children who had the greatest increase in BMI throughout childhood [25]. Faster growth in children is also associated with fat mass in adults in five cohorts from low- and middle-income countries [6]. Given the increasing evidence that childhood obesity is an independent risk factor for CVD, these observations have major implications for the prevention of CVD. However, although the above data strongly support the growth acceleration concept, it remains possible that both rapid growth in childhood and long-term risk of obesity and CVD are a consequence of the same underlying genetic tendency. For example, common genetic variants for adult obesity have been associated with faster weight and length gain in both infancy and childhood [26].

Mechanisms

Despite growing evidence for the developmental origins of adult disease, the underlying mechanisms remain poorly defined. Evidence from animal models and experimental studies in infancy suggest that confounding by environmental and genetic factors is unlikely to explain the impact of early growth/nutrition on later health [9]. However, the exact nature of the exposure in early life, its timing, and the 'coupling mechanisms' that link early nutrition with later health are all poorly understood.

In terms of exposure, it is difficult to separate the programming effects of growth in infancy from those of nutritional factors, such as protein intake, that influence growth. However, the relative importance of growth is supported by evidence from animal models [3, 9] and observations that faster growth is associated with later risk factors for CVD even in infants breastfed [22, 23]. The critical window for the effects of growth/nutrition may extend throughout childhood [25], but includes at least a window in the first year of life, a hypothesis supported by several RCTs [10, 22–24]. In fact, the most sensitive window for programming by infant growth may even be as early as the first few weeks after birth [9].

Two main generic hypotheses have been proposed to explain the 'coupling mechanisms' linking early exposures such as growth with later biological effects such as CVD [as reviewed in 9]. The first, the role of epigenetic changes that persist throughout life, is supported by recent evidence in animal models. Plagemann et al. [27] showed that neonatal overfeeding in rats (which leads to development of the metabolic syndrome later in life) was associated with increased methylation of CpG residues in the insulin receptor promoter gene. Although this epigenetic change did not affect insulin receptor gene expression in the short term, the authors speculated that increased methylation of this allele could predispose to insulin insensitivity under adverse environmental conditions later in life.

The second hypothesis suggests that early growth acceleration permanently affects hormonal axes that regulate bodyweight, food intake and metabolism, and hence fat deposition. Hormonal changes in infancy (possibly via changes to the hypothalamic circuitry regulating appetite) could influence the satiety response and increase food intake throughout life, thereby increasing the risk of obesity and CVD. In support of this, formula feeding and infant-initiated bottle emptying in the first half of infancy was associated with excess weight gain during late infancy [28], while bottle feeding (with either infant formula or human milk), and faster infant weight gain were associated with a lower satiety response later in life [29]. The endocrine changes that allow a resetting of appetite are unknown, but evidence of programming effects of early growth in genetically leptin-deficient ob/ob mice suggests that these effects are independent of leptin [30]. The adverse effects of faster early growth on long-term health are seen in diverse animal species, and so may reflect more fundamental biological processes. As first suggested by McCay [3], early growth may program long-term aging and age-related processes possibly by mechanisms that affect the insulin/IGF-1 systems [9].

Public Health Implications

The idea that modifiable factors in early life can affect the main risk factors for atherosclerosis provides a major opportunity for the primary prevention of CVD. For example, four of the six most common risk factors for mortality in both richer and poorer countries (high blood pressure, obesity, and high blood glucose and cholesterol concentrations; WHO statistics) are influenced by infant nutrition/growth. Furthermore, since early-life factors affect obesity and endocrine changes such as higher IGF-1 concentration, both of which are key risk factors for the development of malignant disease, optimizing nutrition and growth in infancy may have broader benefits for health.

Prevention will be particularly critical for low- and middle-income countries which face the greatest increase in NCDs. Already in every region except Africa, NCDs account for greater mortality than communicable, maternal, perinatal and nutritional conditions combined [1]. This prevalence is projected to increase further by 15% globally between 2010 and 2020, with the greatest increases occurring in Africa, Southeast Asia and the Eastern Mediterranean [1]. Importantly, greater mortality from NCDs in younger individuals (<70 years) in low-income compared to high-income countries disproportionately affects bread winners, and so is predicted to reduce family income, drive up health care costs, and exacerbate poverty. As a consequence, the rapid rise in NCDs even threatens to impede progress on meeting the Millennium Development Goals [1].

However, despite substantial evidence for the impact of infant nutrition on NCDs, public health policy in low-income countries faces several major obstacles to change. Although it is now well accepted that undernutrition in the first 1,000 days after conception has major adverse implications for long-term health and human capital [31], the concept that *overnutrition* in this critical period may also have harmful long-term consequences remains underappreciated. Countries such as India have heterogeneous populations, with many millions at risk of both overnutrition and undernutrition – the so called 'double burden' of disease [32]. Therefore, public health strategies need to be carefully targeted as a 'one size fits all' nutrition policy is unlikely to achieve optimal benefits for health [32]. Furthermore, given rapid changes in lifestyle, by focusing almost exclusively on undernutrition, the nutritional community in many low- and middle-income countries is in danger of fighting 'yesterday's battles'.

Conclusions

The WHO has identified NCDs as the most important global health issue of the 21st century. Consequently, in November 2012, WHO members agreed a global monitoring framework to help prevent NCDs, along with a voluntary target of reducing premature mortality from NCD by 25% by 2025. There is now increasing evidence to suggest that optimizing growth and nutrition in infancy will help achieve these targets.

Disclosure Statement

The author declares that no financial or other conflict of interest exists in relation to the content of the chapter.

References

1 WHO Global status report on non-communicable diseases 2010. Geneva, World Health Organization, 2011.
2 Miranda JJ, Kinra S, Casas JP, et al: Non-communicable diseases in low- and middle-income countries: context, determinants and health policy. Trop Med Int Health 2008;13: 1225–1234.
3 McCay CM: Is longevity compatible with optimum growth? Science 1933;77:410–411.
4 Barker DJP: Fetal origins of coronary heart disease. BMJ 1995;311:171–174.
5 Yang Z, Huffman SL: Nutrition in pregnancy and early childhood and associations with obesity in developing countries. Matern Child Nutr 2013;9(suppl 1):105–119.
6 Kuzawa CW, Hallal PC, Adair L, et al: Birth weight, postnatal weight gain, and adult body composition in five low and middle income countries. Am J Hum Biol 2012;24:5–13.
7 Hawkesworth S: Exploiting dietary supplementation trials to assess the impact of prenatal environment on CVD risk. Proc Nutr Soc 2009;68:78–88.
8 Vaidya A, Saville N, Shrestha BP, et al: Effects of antenatal multiple micronutrient supplementation on children's weight and size at 2 years of age in Nepal: follow-up of a double-blind randomized controlled trial. Lancet 2008;371:492–499.
9 Singhal A: Does early growth affect long-term risk factors for cardiovascular disease? in Lucas A, Makrides M, Ziegler EE (eds): Importance of growth for Health and Development. Nestlé Nutr Inst Workshop Ser Pediatr Program. Vevey, Nestec/Basel, Karger, 2010, vol 65, pp 55–69.
10 Singhal A, Cole TJ, Lucas A: Early nutrition in preterm infants and later blood pressure: two cohorts after randomised trials. Lancet 2001;357:413–419.

11 Singhal A, Lucas A: Early origins of cardio-vascular disease. Is there a unifying hypothesis? Lancet 2004;363:1642–1645.

12 Beyerlein A, Von Kries R: Breastfeeding and body composition in children: will there ever be conclusive empirical evidence for a protective effect against overweight. Am J Clin Nutr 2011;94(suppl):1772S–1775S.

13 Fewtrell MS: The evidence for public health recommendations on infant feeding. Early Human Development 2011;87:715–721.

14 Gale C, Logan KM, Santhakumaran S, et al: Effect of breastfeeding compared with formula feeding on infant body composition: a systematic review and meta-analysis. Am J Clin Nutr 2012;95:656–669.

15 Weng SF, Redsell SA, Swift JA, et al: Systematic review and meta-analyses of risk factors for childhood overweight identifiable during infancy. Arch Dis Child DOI: 10.1136/arch-dischild-2012-302963.

16 Brion MJ, Lawlor DA, Matijasevich A, et al: What are the causal effects of breastfeeding on IQ, obesity and blood pressure? Evidence from comparing high-income with middle-income cohorts. Int J Epidemiol 2011;40: 670–680.

17 Ozanne SE, Hales CN: Catch-up growth and obesity in male mice. Nature 2004;427:411–412.

18 Kramer MS, Matush L, Vanilovich I, et al: Effects of prolonged and exclusive breastfeeding on child height, weight, adiposity, and blood pressure at age 6.5 years: evidence from a large randomized trial. Am J Clin Nutr 2007;86:1717–1721.

19 Singhal A, Lanigan J: Breast-feeding, early growth and later obesity. Obesity Rev 2007;8: 51–54.

20 Monteiro POA, Victora CG: Rapid growth in infancy and childhood and obesity in later life – a systematic review. Obesity Rev 2005;6: 143–154.

21 Fall CH, Sachdev HS, Osmond C, et al: Adult metabolic syndrome and impaired glucose tolerance are associated with different patterns of BMI gain during infancy: data from the New Delhi Birth Cohort. Diabetes Care 2008;31:2349–2356.

22 Singhal A, Cole TJ, Fewtrell M, et al: Promotion of faster weight gain in infants born small for gestational age: is there an adverse effect on later blood pressure? Circulation 2007;115:213–220.

23 Singhal A, Kennedy K, Lanigan J, et al: Nutrition in infancy and long-term risk of obesity: evidence from two randomised controlled trials. Am J Clin Nutr 2010;92:1133–1144.

24 Koletzko B, von Kries R, Monasterolo R, et al: Lower protein in infant formula is associated with lower weight up to age 2 y: a randomized clinical trial. Am J Clin Nutr 2009;89: 1–10.

25 Bhargava SK, Sachdev HS, Fall CHD, et al: Relation of serial changes in childhood body mass index to impaired glucose tolerance in young adulthood. N Engl J Med 2004;350: 865–875.

26 Elks CE, Loos RJF, Hardy R, et al: Adult obesity variants are associated with greater childhood weight gain and a faster tempo of growth: the 1946 British Birth Cohort Study. Am J Clin Nutr 2012;95:1150–1156.

27 Plagemann A, Roepke K, Harder T, et al: Epigenetic malprogramming of the insulin receptor promoter due to developmental overfeeding. J Perinat Med 2010;38:393–400.

28 Li R, Fein SB, Grummer-Strawn LM: Association of breast-feeding intensity and bottle-emptying behaviors at early infancy with infants' risk for excess weight at late infancy. Pediatrics 2008;122:S77–S84.

29 DiSantis KI, Collins BN, Fisher JO, et al: Do infants fed directly from the breast have improved appetite regulation and slower growth compared with infants fed from a bottle. Int J Behav Nutr Phys Act 2011;8:89–100.

30 Cottrell EC, Martin-Gronert MS, Fernandez-Twinn DS, et al: Leptin-independent programming of adult body weight and adiposity in mice. Endocrinology 2011;152:476–482.

31 Jain V, Singhal A: Catch up growth in low birth weight infants: striking a healthy balance. Rev Endocr Metab Disord 2012;13: 141–147.

32 Victora CG, Adair L, Fall C, et al: Maternal and child undernutrition: consequences for adult health and human capital. Lancet 2008; 371:340–357.

Future Perspectives: Impact of Early Life Nutrition

Black RE, Singhal A, Uauy R (eds): International Nutrition: Achieving Millennium Goals and Beyond.
Nestlé Nutr Inst Workshop Ser, vol 78, pp 133–140, (DOI: 10.1159/000354952)
Nestec Ltd., Vevey/S. Karger AG., Basel, © 2014

Obesity and the Metabolic Syndrome in Developing Countries: Focus on South Asians

Anoop Misra[a–d] · Swati Bhardwaj[b–d]

[a]Fortis C-DOC Center of Excellence for Diabetes, Metabolic Diseases and Endocrinology,
[b]National Diabetes, Obesity and Cholesterol Foundation, [c]Diabetes Foundation (India), and
[d]Center for Nutrition and Metabolic Research, New Delhi, India

Abstract

With improvement in the economic situation, an increasing prevalence of obesity and the metabolic syndrome is seen in developing countries in South Asia. Particularly vulnerable population groups include women and children, and intra-country and inter-country migrants. The main causes are increasing urbanization, nutrition transition, reduced physical activity, and genetic predisposition. Some evidence suggests that widely prevalent perinatal undernutrition and childhood 'catch-up' obesity may play a role in adult-onset metabolic syndrome and type 2 diabetes. Data show that atherogenic dyslipidemia, glucose intolerance, thrombotic tendency, subclinical inflammation, and endothelial dysfunction are higher in South Asians than white Caucasians. Many of these manifestations are more severe even at an early age in South Asians than white Caucasians. Metabolic and cardiovascular risks in South Asians are also heightened by their higher body fat, truncal subcutaneous fat, intra-abdominal fat, and ectopic fat deposition (liver fat, muscle fat, etc.). Further, cardiovascular risk cluster manifests at a lower level of adiposity and abdominal obesity. The cutoffs of body mass index and waist circumference for defining obesity and abdominal obesity, respectively, have been lowered for Asians, and same has been endorsed for South Asians in the UK. The economic cost of obesity and related diseases in developing countries, having meager health budget, is enormous. Increasing awareness of these noncommunicable diseases and how to prevent them should be focus of population-wide prevention strategies in South Asian developing countries. Community intervention programs focusing on increased physical activity and healthier food options for schoolchildren are urgently required. Data from such a major intervention program conducted by us on adolescent urban schoolchildren in north India (project MARG) have shown encouraging results and could serve as a model for initiating such programs in other South Asian developing countries.

Developing countries, particularly South Asia, are witnessing a rapid increase seen in type 2 diabetes mellitus (T2DM) and coronary heart disease (CHD) [1]. During the previous three decades, the prevalence of T2DM has doubled in India. Insulin resistance and clustering of other proatherogenic factors (the metabolic syndrome), frequently seen in South Asians, are important contributory factors for T2DM and CHD [2].

Rapid demographic, nutritional, and economic changes are occurring in South Asians [1]. The life expectancy and percentage of elderly population have increased. Most importantly, globalization of diets and consumption of nontraditional 'fast-foods' have occurred at a rapid pace in urban areas. Furthermore, these dietary changes are most noticeable in children. In South Asian countries, rapid increase in western fast-food outlets, sale of aerated sweet drinks and increased consumption of fried snacks in school children are being commonly seen [3]. In addition, South Asians are less physically active, and sedentary lifestyle is increasing, particularly in children [1, 4]. Further, migration from villages to cities is increasing. These intra-country migrants become urbanized, mechanized, resulting in nutritional imbalance, physical inactivity, stress, and increased consumption of alcohol and tobacco [5].

Nationally representative studies regarding the prevalence of the metabolic syndrome are generally not available from any South Asian country. Available data indicate that the prevalence of the metabolic syndrome in Asian Indians varies according to region, extent of urbanization, lifestyle patterns and socio-economic/cultural factors [1–2, 6–8]. Recent data show that about one third of the urban population in large cities in India has the metabolic syndrome [1]. The interaction of various factors which could contribute to insulin resistance, diabetes, and CHD is shown in figure 1.

The phenotype of obesity and body fat distribution are distinctive in South Asians and are important contributory factors in the development of insulin resistance and the metabolic syndrome [1–2, 9]. Key points have been summarized below.

1 Average body mass index (BMI) value in South Asians is lower than that seen in white Caucasians, Mexican-Americans and Blacks. However, BMI in Asian Indians increases as they become affluent and urbanized [1, 2].

2 South Asians have a high percentage of body fat as compared to white Caucasians and Blacks, despite lower average BMI values, which is partly explained by body build (trunk-to-leg length ratio and slenderness),

Misra · Bhardwaj

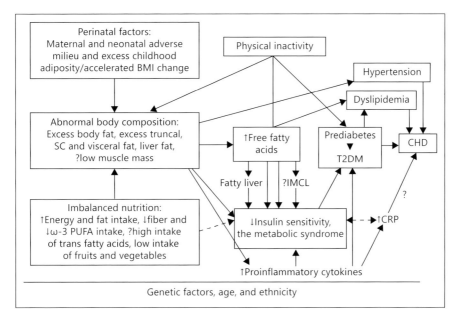

Fig. 1. Complex interactions of genetic, perinatal, nutritional and other acquired factors in development of insulin resistance, T2DM and CHD in Asian Indians. PUFA = Polyunsaturated fatty acid; CRP = C-reactive protein; IMCL = intramyocellular lipids; SC = subcutaneous.

muscularity, adaptation to chronic calorie deprivation, and ethnicity. Higher body fat seen in South Asians than Caucasians at similar BMI was clearly demonstrable in Asian Indians based in Singapore who showed BMI to be 3 lower than white Caucasians at any given percentage of body fat [1–2, 10].

3   Importantly, morbidities related to excess adiposity (diabetes, hypertension, dyslipidemia) occur more frequently at lower BMI levels in Asians than in white Caucasians [1, 10].

4   High prevalence of abdominal obesity has been reported in South Asians by several investigators, and is also seen in Asian Indians with BMI <25 [6, 10–12]. Further, although the average waist circumference in South Asians appears to be lower, abdominal adiposity as measured by computerized axial topography is significantly more than in white Caucasians [10]. Based on these data, classification of obesity has been revised for Asian Indians (table 1) [13, 14]. These cutoffs have been endorsed for South Asians in UK recently [15].

5   Intra-abdominal adipose tissue in South Asians is comparatively more than white Caucasians [9, 10, 12].

6   Truncal subcutaneous adipose tissue (measured by subscapular and supra-iliac skinfolds) is thicker in South Asians than white Caucasians (in both

Table 1. Consensus guidelines for defining obesity, abdominal obesity and the metabolic syndrome in Asian Indians, adapted from Misra et al. [13]

Generalized obesity (BMI[1] cutoffs)	Abdominal obesity (waist circumference cutoffs)	The metabolic syndrome[2]
Normal: 18.0–22.9 Overweight: 23.0–24.9 Obesity: >25	Men: ≥90 cm Women: ≥80 cm	Abdominal obesity: waist circumference cutoffs as defined in previous column (nonobligatory) Blood glucose: ≥100 mg/dl Hypertension: ≥130/≥85 mm Hg Triglycerides: ≥150 mg/dl HDL-C: males <40 mg/dl, females <50 mg/dl

[1] Calculated as kg/m^2.
[2] No parameter is obligatory; three out of five need to be present to diagnose the metabolic syndrome.

adults and children), correlating more closely with insulin resistance than intra-abdominal adipose tissue [1].

7 The fat is deposited in excess in 'ectopic sites': skeletal muscles, liver, etc. The latter is comparatively higher in Asian Indians as compared to white Caucasians and correlates with insulin resistance [10]. This appears to have strong genetic influence [16–20].

8 Finally, South Asians appear to be 'metabolically obese', though BMI levels may fall into the category of 'nonobese'. This phenomenon is partially explained by excess body fat, high intra-abdominal and subcutaneous fat, and ectopic fat deposition in various organs and body sites, which may contribute to insulin resistance, dyslipidemia, hyperglycemia, and excess procoagulant factors in South Asians [1, 21].

Prevention and Control of Obesity and the Metabolic Syndrome in South Asians

Prevention of these conditions requires early and aggressive management based on the following key principles.

1 Intensive efforts should be made to make South Asians aware that they are at higher risk for development of T2DM and CHD than other ethnic groups.

2 Preventive measures should be particularly vigorous for those with the family history of T2DM or premature CHD.

3 Adequate nutrition during the intrauterine period should be given to prevent early-life adverse events, which may promote insulin resistance in adulthood.

4 Therapeutic lifestyle changes should be encouraged from childhood, with strict advice of regular physical activity and restricted use of television/Internet usage. According to the recent guidelines for Asian Indians, children should undertake at least 60 min of outdoor physical activity. Screen time (television/computers) should be less than 2 h a day. Healthy lifestyle should be inculcated in children through rigorous implementation of school health programs.

5 Physicians should strictly monitor velocity of growth of children to avoid childhood obesity and 'catch-up obesity'.

6 Bodyweight and anthropometric indexes for adults should be maintained within normal limits based on the recent data. According to recent consensus statement for Asian Indians, BMI should be maintained between 18 and 22.9, and waist circumference should be maintained below 90 cm for men and 80 cm for women [13].

7 Overweight individuals and those with abdominal obesity should be actively managed to lose weight by lifestyle measures [22, 23].

8 Detection of one component of the metabolic syndrome should lead to search for the other components and its management [13].

9 In general, a total of 60 min daily of physical activity is recommended for prevention and management of obesity and the metabolic syndrome for Asian Indians according to recently approved guidelines. This includes aerobic activity, work-related activity and muscle-strengthening activity [23].

10 Diets should be balanced containing carbohydrate (55–65% of calories) with emphasis on complex carbohydrates, restricted total fats and saturated fat (7–10% of the total calories), adequate MUFAs, ω-3 PUFAs and fiber. Trans fatty acid-containing oils and foods should be strictly avoided [22].

11 Research on insulin resistance and the metabolic syndrome in South Asians should be targeted on the following:

   a Prevalence of the metabolic syndrome in various South-Asian countries.

   b Etiological factors of insulin resistance, particularly studies on genetics and genetic-environmental interaction.

   c Associations of specific macro- and micronutrients in South Asian diet with insulin resistance (e.g. ω-3 PUFAs and dietary fiber).

d The relationship with novel cardiovascular risk factors (e.g. high-sensitivity C-reactive protein).
e Intervention with insulin sensitizers and other drugs.
f Diagnostic criteria of the metabolic syndrome and morbidity correlation in children.
g Effective health intervention methods of imparting lifestyle and diet-related health messages in children.

Community Intervention Programs for Childhood Obesity in India

Community-based interventions are aimed at generating awareness and providing a conducive environment for children to follow a healthy lifestyle (balanced diet and increased physical activity) and promote healthy food alternatives. In India, we have initiated comprehensive programs aiming at childhood obesity, namely CHETNA (Hindi for 'The Awareness'; Children Health Education through Nutrition and Health Awareness program), which was carried out in new Delhi, and MARG (Hindi for 'The Path'; Medical Education for Children/Adolescents for Realistic Prevention of Obesity and Diabetes and for Healthy Ageing), carried out in 15 cities of North India covering nearly 700,000 children. Under these programs, children are given nutritional and physical activity education with the help of lectures, leaflets, debates and skits. These comprehensive programs initiated on a large scale for the first time in South Asia aimed to impart education regarding healthy lifestyle not only to children, but also to teachers and parents. The MARG program is the first large-scale community intervention project in South Asia which focuses 100% on primary prevention of not only diabetes, but on noncommunicable diseases in general [24–32].

Disclosure Statement

The authors have no conflict of interest.

References

1 Misra A, Khurana L: Obesity and the metabolic syndrome in developing countries. J Clin Endocrinol Metab 2008;93:S9–S30.
2 Misra A, Vikram NK: Insulin resistance syndrome (metabolic syndrome) and obesity in Asian Indians: evidence and implications. Nutrition 2004;20:482–491.
3 Misra A, Khurana L, Isharwal S, Bhardwaj S: South Asian diets and insulin resistance. Br J Nutr 2009;101:465–473.
4 Bedi US, Singh S, Syed A, et al: Coronary artery disease in South Asians: an emerging risk group. Cardiol Rev 2006;14:74–80.

Misra · Bhardwaj

5 Misra A, Ganda OP: Migration and its impact on adiposity and type 2 diabetes. Nutrition 2007;23:696–708.
6 Vikram NK, Pandey RM, Misra A, et al: Non-obese (BMI <25) Asian Indians with normal waist circumference have high cardiovascular risk. Nutrition 2003;19:503–509.
7 Ramachandran A, Snehalatha C, Satyavani K, et al: Metabolic syndrome in urban Asian Indian adults – a population study using modified ATP III criteria. Diabetes Res Clin Pract 2003;60:199–204.
8 Gupta R, Deedwania PC, Gupta A, et al: Prevalence of metabolic syndrome in an Indian urban population. Int J Cardiol 2004;97:257–261.
9 Deurenberg P, Yap M, van Staveren WA: Body mass index and percent body fat: a meta analysis among different ethnic groups. Int J Obes Relat Metab Disord 1998;22:1164–1171.
10 Misra A, Vikram NK: Clinical and patho-physiological consequences of abdominal adiposity and abdominal adipose tissue depots. Nutrition 2003;19:457–466.
11 Dudeja V, Misra A, Pandey RM, et al: BMI does not accurately predict overweight in Asian Indians in northern India. Br J Nutr 2001;86:105–112.
12 Chandalia M, Lin P, Seenivasan T, et al: Insulin resistance and body fat distribution in South Asian men compared to Caucasian men. PLoS One 2007;2:e812.
13 Misra A, Chowbey PK, Makkar BM, et al: Consensus statement for diagnosis of obesity, abdominal obesity and the metabolic syndrome for Asian Indians and recommendations for physical activity, medical and surgical management. J Assoc Physicians India 2009;57:163–170.
14 WHO Expert Consultation: Appropriate body-mass index for Asian populations and its implications for policy and intervention strategies. Lancet 2004;363:157–163.
15 Tougher obesity measure set for British Asian. http://www.business-standard.com/article/pti-stories/tougher-obesity-measure-set-for-british-asian-113070300615_1.html (assessed 17th July 2013).
16 Bhatt SP, Nigam P, Misra A, et al: Genetic variation in the patatin-like phospholipase domain-containing protein-3 (PNPLA-3) gene in Asian Indians with nonalcoholic fatty liver disease. Metab Syndr Relat Disord 2013, E-pub ahead of print.
17 Bhatt SP, Nigam P, Misra A, et al: Association of peroxisome proliferator activated receptor-γ gene with non-alcoholic fatty liver disease in Asian Indians residing in north India. Gene 2013;512:143–147.
18 Bhatt SP, Nigam P, Misra A, et al: Association of the Myostatin gene with obesity, abdominal obesity and low lean body mass and in non-diabetic Asian Indians in north India. PLoS One 2012;7:e40977.
19 Bhatt SP, Misra A, Sharma M, et al: Ala/Ala genotype of Pro12Ala polymorphism in the peroxisome proliferator-activated receptor-γ2 gene is associated with obesity and insulin resistance in Asian Indians. Diabetes Technol Ther 2012;14:828–834.
20 Bhatt SP, Nigam P, Misra A, et al: SREBP-2 1784 G/C genotype is associated with non-alcoholic fatty liver disease in north Indians. Dis Markers 2011;31:371–377.
21 Misra A, Shrivastava U: Obesity and dyslipidemia in South Asians. Nutrients 2013;5:2708–2733.
22 Misra A, Nigam P, Hills AP, et al, Physical Activity Consensus Group: Consensus physical activity guidelines for Asian Indians. Diabetes Technol Ther 2012;14:83–98.
23 Misra A, Sharma R, Gulati S, et al, National Dietary Guidelines Consensus Group: Consensus dietary guidelines for healthy living and prevention of obesity, the metabolic syndrome, diabetes, and related disorders in Asian Indians. Diabetes Technol Ther 2011;13:683–694.
24 Gupta N, Shah P, Nayyar S, Misra A: Childhood obesity and the metabolic syndrome in developing countries. Indian J Pediatr 2013;80(suppl 1):S28–S37.
25 Bhardwaj S, Misra A, Khurana L, et al: Childhood obesity in Asian Indians: a burgeoning cause of insulin resistance, diabetes and subclinical inflammation. Asia Pac J Clin Nutr 2008;17(suppl 1):172–175.
26 Gupta N, Goel K, Shah P, Misra A: Childhood obesity in developing countries: epidemiology, determinants, and prevention. Endocr Rev 2012;33:48–70.
27 Misra A, Shah P, Goel K, et al: The high burden of obesity and abdominal obesity in urban Indian schoolchildren: a multicentric study of 38,296 children. Ann Nutr Metab 2011;58:203–211.

28 Gupta DK, Shah P, Misra A, et al: Secular trends in prevalence of overweight and obesity from 2006 to 2009 in urban Asian Indian adolescents aged 14–17 years. PLoS One 2011;6:e17221.

29 Singhal N, Misra A, Shah P, et al: Impact of intensive school-based nutrition education and lifestyle interventions on insulin resistance, β-cell function, disposition index, and subclinical inflammation among Asian Indian adolescents: a controlled intervention study. Metab Syndr Relat Disord 2011;9:143–150.

30 Gupta N, Shah P, Goel K, et al: Imbalanced dietary profile, anthropometry, and lipids in urban Asian Indian adolescents and young adults. J Am Coll Nutr 2010;29:81–91.

31 Shah P, Misra A, Gupta N, et al: Improvement in nutrition-related knowledge and behaviour of urban Asian Indian school children: findings from the 'Medical education for children/Adolescents for Realistic prevention of obesity and diabetes and for healthy aGeing' (MARG) intervention study. Br J Nutr 2010;104:427–436.

32 Singhal N, Misra A, Shah P, et al: Secular trends in obesity, regional adiposity and metabolic parameters among Asian Indian adolescents in north India: a comparative data analysis of two selective samples 5 years apart (2003, 2008). Ann Nutr Metab 2010;56:176–181.

Black RE, Singhal A, Uauy R (eds): International Nutrition: Achieving Millennium Goals and Beyond.
Nestlé Nutr Inst Workshop Ser, vol 78, pp 141–153, (DOI: 10.1159/000354954)
Nestec Ltd., Vevey/S. Karger AG., Basel, © 2014

Preventing Atopy and Allergic Disease

Ralf G. Heine

Department of Allergy and Immunology, Royal Children's Hospital, Murdoch Children's Research
Institute, University of Melbourne, Melbourne, VIC, Australia

Abstract

Due to the recent exponential increase in food allergies and atopic disorders, effective allergy prevention has become a public health priority in many developed regions. Important preventive strategies include the promotion of breastfeeding and vaginal deliveries, judicious use of perinatal antibiotics, as well as the avoidance of maternal tobacco smoking. Breastfeeding for at least 6 months and introduction of complementary solids from 4–6 months are generally recommended. Complex oligosaccharides in breast milk support the establishment of bifidobacteria in the neonatal gut which stimulate regulatory T lymphocyte responses and enhance tolerance development. Maternal elimination diets during pregnancy or lactation are not effective in preventing allergies. If exclusive breastfeeding is not possible, (supplemental) feeding with a partially hydrolyzed whey-based formula or extensively hydrolyzed casein-based formula may reduce the risk of cow's milk allergy and atopic dermatitis in infants with a family history of atopy. By contrast, asthma and allergic rhinitis at 4–6 years of age are not prevented by this approach. Soy formula and amino acid-based formula have no proven role in allergy prevention. Perinatal supplementation with probiotics and/or prebiotics may reduce the risk of atopic dermatitis, but no reliable effect on the prevention of food allergy or respiratory allergies has so far been found. A randomized trial on maternal fish oil supplementation during pregnancy found that atopic dermatitis and egg sensitization in the first year of life were significantly reduced, but no preventive effect for food allergies was demonstrated. The role of vitamin D deficiency or excess as a risk factor for food allergy and atopic disorders requires further study.
© 2014 Nestec Ltd., Vevey/S. Karger AG, Basel

Introduction

Over the past two decades, the prevalence of allergic disorders has increased exponentially [1]. This trend has mainly affected Western societies but is now also evident in emerging economies in the Asia-Pacific region [2, 3]. The greatest increase in allergic disorders has involved food allergy and atopic eczema in infants and young children, whereas the incidences of asthma and respiratory allergies appear to have stabilized. From 1995 to 2005, hospital admissions in Australia for food anaphylaxis have increased by about 350% [4], and the rate of challenge-proven food allergy has risen to more than 10% in 1-year-old children (peanut 3.0%, egg 8.9%) [5]. In view of this recent sharp increase in allergic disorders, effective allergy prevention strategies have become a major public health priority. Primary allergy prevention seeks to minimize the risk of allergic sensitization to foods and environmental allergens. Several approaches to allergy prevention have been developed (table 1). Strategies range from attempts to modify exposures to pollutants (e.g. tobacco smoke), dietary measures (e.g. promotion of breastfeeding) or modification of microbial exposures (e.g. reduced use of perinatal antibiotics).

The recent surge in allergic diseases has coincided with improved sanitation and a reduction in infectious diseases *('hygiene hypothesis')*. However, the etiology of allergic disorders is not completely understood. While genetic risk factors for allergic disease are well recognized (e.g. filaggrin gene defects in atopic dermatitis [6], thymic stromal lymphopoietin polymorphisms in asthma [7] or eosinophilic esophagitis [8]), these alone cannot explain the recent increase in allergic diseases. It appears more likely that environmental factors associated with a 'Western lifestyle' (e.g. environmental pollutants, microbial burden and dietary factors) modify genetic allergic risk and gene expression. The role of epigenetic imprinting in this process has been highlighted [9, 10]. Tobacco smoking is another well-recognized factor that stimulates T helper 2 lymphocyte responses and increases the allergic risk in young infants [11]. Avoidance of maternal tobacco smoking during pregnancy and lactation is therefore a key strategy in minimizing allergy risk.

Early Gut Colonization, Microbial Biodiversity and Allergy Risk

During early infancy and childhood, the fecal microbiome undergoes important developmental changes. These changes are thought to impact significantly on the maturation of immune responses and on tolerance development. The sterile and initially aerobic gut environment of the neonate is first colonized by facultative bacteria, including *Escherichia coli*, *Enterococcus* spp. and *Staphylococcus* spp.

Table 1. Examples of dietary strategies for primary allergy prevention

Promotion of exclusive breastfeeding to at least 6 months of age
Introduction of complementary diet from 4 to 6 months of age
Maternal fish oil supplementation during pregnancy
Maternal probiotic/prebiotic supplementation during pregnancy and lactation
Use of partially or extensively hydrolyzed formula (if breastfeeding is not possible)
Probiotic/prebiotic supplementation of maternal diet or infant formula

[12, 13]. Complex oligosaccharides in breast milk provide the substrate which promotes the establishment of anaerobic bacteria, including *Bifidobacterium*, *Bacteroides* and *Clostridium* spp. Bifidobacteria are thought to be crucial in promoting mucosal tolerance via the stimulation of innate immune responses (Toll-like receptors) and induction of regulatory T lymphocyte responses [14, 15]. The mode of delivery affects the composition of the fecal microbiota in the newborn period. In infants born via Caesarean section, the gut microbiota reflect the maternal skin flora, including Staphylococci, rather than vaginal flora that predominates in infants born via vaginal tract delivery [16]. The differences in early gut colonization between vaginally and surgically delivered infants have profound effects on early tolerance development. It is therefore not surprising that infants born via Caesarean section have a higher risk of allergic disease and asthma [17, 18]. By contrast, term infants who were born vaginally and were breastfed exclusively seem to have the most 'beneficial' gut microbiota (highest numbers of bifidobacteria and lowest numbers of *Clostridium difficile* and *E. coli*) [19].

Strategies to Promote Fecal Microbial Biodiversity

Gut microbiota and environmental microbial burden play a central role in early immune development and are likely to influence immunological events that lead to allergy. For example, growing up in a rural farm environment has been shown to significantly reduce the risk of asthma and allergic disease in children [10, 20]. There are significant differences in the gut microbiota profiles between allergic and nonallergic infants and children. Allergy and asthma risk are inversely associated with the degree of microbial biodiversity [21, 22]. Infants with IgE-associated eczema have significantly reduced fecal microbial diversity in the first month of life, compared to nonatopic infants [23, 24]. Modification of early gut colonization and fecal microbial diversity in infancy may thus provide an avenue for preventive or therapeutic strategies. Possible ways to establish a tolerogenic gut milieu in early infancy include the promotion of natural vaginal deliveries, exclusive breastfeeding for at least 6 months, judicious use of perinatal antibiot-

Table 2. Factors associated with early gut colonization

Mode of delivery
Type of infant feeding
Gestational age
Infant hospitalization
Antibiotic use
Urban/rural environment

ics and living in a farm environment (table 2). Probiotic or prebiotic supplementation has also been shown to modify the risk of allergies, particularly for atopic dermatitis in infancy [25, 26].

Dietary Allergy Prevention

Breastfeeding is one of the main pillars in allergy prevention [27–31]. Breast milk provides the most appropriate source of nutrition for the young infant as it contains a species-specific mixture of nutrients, growth factors and protective maternal antibodies. The World Health Organization (WHO) recommends exclusive breastfeeding for at least 6 months, taking into consideration not only allergy prevention but also general nutritional aspects, including prevention of respiratory and gastrointestinal infection. Breastfeeding is associated with the establishment of fecal microbiota high in bifidobacteria [32]. Bifidobacteria are thought to promote mucosal tolerance interact via regulatory T lymphocytes and Toll-like receptors [14]. The duration of exclusive breastfeeding appears to influence the risk of allergic disease [33, 34]. The protective effect of breastfeeding on eczema in the first 2 years of life appears to be modified by maternal allergy status [35]. Several studies have found no evidence that exclusive breastfeeding for 6 months or more prevented asthma, eczema or atopy at 5 years of age [31, 36]. In addition, a recent large longitudinal study showed that exclusive breastfeeding for at least 3 months was associated with a protective effect against infantile eczema, asthma and food allergies at 7 years of age, but a paradoxically increased asthma risk later in life [37].

Hydrolyzed Formulas

Partially hydrolyzed formula (PHF) has been recommended for allergy prevention in infants with a family history [30]. This recommendation follows the Cochrane review on the role of hydrolyzed formula in allergy prevention which found a limited beneficial effect (compared to cow's milk formula; CMF) in infants with a family history of atopy [38]. The German Infant Nutritional Intervention (GINI) study [39], to date the largest quasi-randomized trial comparing the effects of PHF, extensively hydrolyzed formula (EHF) and CMF, has provided the most convincing data for a protective effect for PHF and EHF. However, other studies have found no significant preventive effect for PHF [40]. The GINI study demonstrated a sustained preventive effect against atopic eczema until the age of 6 years after use of whey-based PHF or casein-based EHF, but no effect on respiratory allergies and asthma. A meta-analysis has confirmed a treatment benefit for PHF in infants with atopic dermatitis [41]. Health economic modeling found this approach cost-effective in a range of health care settings [42–44]. Others have questioned the role PHF and cautioned against overstating the preventive effect for allergic disease [40, 45]. In summary, hydrolyzed formulas may prevent atopic dermatitis in high-risk infants, but respiratory allergies are not prevented.

Soy Formula

In past years, there has been a growing concern about the safety of exclusive soy feeding in infants under 6 months, as reflected in a position paper by the European Society for Pediatric Gastroenterology and Nutrition [46]. A Cochrane review based on three randomized clinical trials showed no significant preventive effect of soy formula on the development of allergic disease [47]. Although soy formula may have a role in the treatment of cow's milk allergy (CMA), as well as conditions such as lactose intolerance or galactosemia, its use for the purpose of allergy prevention in infants less than 6 months of age is currently not recommended [48].

Amino Acid-Based Formula

Amino acid-based formula (AAF) has been shown to be effective and nutritionally complete in the treatment of infants with CMA [49]. Its preventive effects on food allergy or atopic disorders, however, have never been assessed [28]. This is mainly because the cost of the formula prohibits its widespread use in allergy prevention. In theory, AAF may also have disadvantages in immune maturation of the young infants, as oral tolerance development is believed to be an active regulatory process that requires the stimulation of the infant's gut-associated immune system by ingested antigens [50]. The use of AAF for primary allergy prevention is not recommended.

Timing of the Introduction of Weaning Foods

Fergusson et al. [51] were among the first to demonstrate an increase in risk of atopic dermatitis if weaning solids were introduced before 4 months of age. A large German birth cohort study [52], however, found no protective effect of the delayed introduction (after 4 months) of solids on atopic dermatitis at 4 years of age. Previously, the delayed introduction of common food allergens (cow's milk after 12 months, egg after 2 years and peanut after 3 years) was recommended in an attempt to prevent food allergy [53]. However, more recently there has been a shift away from prolonged avoidance to earlier dietary introduction [54]. Findings from several small studies provide support for the concept of a 'window period' for tolerance induction, whereby tolerance is more likely to be achieved if weaning solids are introduced between 4 and 6 months of age. This reflects the feeding practices in many European countries but is not supported by the current WHO guidelines. Several prospective studies are currently underway to assess the effect of the early complementary diet on allergy risk. Until these studies are available, it will be difficult to make meaningful recommendations regarding the best timing of a complementary diet.

Maternal Elimination Diets during Pregnancy and Lactation

Exposure of the infants to intact food allergens that are secreted into breast milk can be reduced by maternal dietary avoidance [55]. It appeared therefore plausible that modification of diet during pregnancy and lactation may modify allergy risk. The Isle of Wight prevention study [56] examined the effect of breastfeeding (while mothers maintained an allergen-reduced elimination diet), complementary feeding with EHF and concurrent house dust mite avoidance on the development of food allergy and atopy. Although at 2 years the rate of food allergy in the active intervention group was lower, this difference was lost on repeated measurement analysis at 8 years of age. The Cochrane review found no significant primary preventive effect of maternal elimination diets for allergic diseases but warns against possible adverse nutritional outcomes for mother and infant [57]. Maternal elimination diets during lactation may reduce the severity of established eczema (secondary and tertiary prevention). However, maternal elimination diets during pregnancy for the purpose of primary allergy prevention are not deemed effective.

Probiotics and Prebiotics

Infants with allergies have been shown to have significantly lower numbers of fecal bifidobacteria compared to healthy infants [58]. Allergy prevention via supplementation with lactobacilli and bifidobacteria therefore appeared promising. Probiotics and prebiotics have since become of the main strategies in allergy prevention in young infants.

Probiotics

The increase in allergic disorders has commonly been explained by a lack of early microbial stimulation of the immature immune system. The effects are mediated via the innate immune system (Toll-like receptors), resulting in the promotion of T helper 1 differentiation, production of regulatory cytokines (IL-10 and TGF-β) and enhanced intestinal IgA responses [59]. Several studies have demonstrated that perinatal administration of probiotics to mothers in the last weeks of pregnancy and to infants in the first few months of life was associated with a significant reduction in atopic eczema [25, 26, 60]. Nevertheless, results have been varied, depending on the probiotic strain, dose, timing and food matrix used. A study using *Lactobacillus acidophilus* (LAVRI A1) showed a paradoxical increase in allergic sensitization [61]. These studies highlight that outcomes depend considerably on the specific probiotic strains used. The role of probiotics in allergy prevention requires further study [62].

Prebiotics

Complex nondigestible, prebiotic oligosaccharides contained in breast milk provide the unique substrate for bifidobacteria. Infant formulas are usually devoid of such prebiotic oligosaccharides [63]. In recent years, manufactured long-chain fructo-oligosaccharides (FOS) and short-chain galacto-oligosaccharides (GOS) have been added to infant formulas and weaning solids. GOS and FOS promote fecal bifidobacteria in formula-fed infants [64, 65]. A randomized study examined the effects of a FOS/GOS-supplemented hydrolyzed formula on atopic eczema in 259 formula-fed infants during the first 6 months of life [66]. In the study, the FOS/GOS group had significantly lower rates of eczema than the placebo group, but eczema severity was similar for both treatment arms. A more recent European multicenter randomized controlled trial assessed the effect of prebiotics in healthy, low-risk infants from 8 weeks to 12 months [67].

Infants were randomized to standard infant formula supplemented with GOS, FOS and pectin-derived acidic oligosaccharides (n = 414) versus unsupplemented standard formula (n = 416). Prebiotics reduced the incidence of atopic dermatitis by 44% at 12 months, although disease severity was not affected. The number needed to treat in order to prevent one case of atopic dermatitis was 25 infants. Further studies are needed to assess the role of prebiotics in allergy prevention [68].

Immune-Modulating Micronutrients

Several immune-modulating micronutrients are of potential relevance in the prevention of food allergy, including omega-3 long-chain polyunsaturated fatty acids (LC-PUFA; fish oil) and vitamin D.

Omega-3 Long-Chain Polyunsaturated Fatty Acids

Maternal diets high in omega-3 LC-PUFAs are thought to have a protective effect against the development of allergies in the newborn [69]. Supplementation with docosahexaenoic acid (DHA) and eicosapentaenoic acid (EPA) during pregnancy has been shown to increase LC-PUFA concentrations in breast milk [70]. A large randomized clinical trial of maternal fish oil supplementation during pregnancy demonstrated a significant decrease in cord blood concentrations of Th-2 cytokines (IL-4 and IL-13) as well as increased levels of oral tolerance-inducing TGF-β [71]. Palmer et al. [72] assessed the effect of high-dose fish oil supplementation in high-risk infants (i.e. family history of atopy). Infants were randomized to receive either 800 mg DHA plus 100 mg EPA (n = 368), or vegetable oil (n = 338). Supplements were administered to pregnant mothers from 21 weeks' gestation until delivery. Infants were followed to 12 months of age and assessed for allergies by blood and skin testing. Primary outcomes were eczema and food sensitization. Infants in the fish oil-supplemented group had significantly lower rates of atopic eczema (7 vs. 12%; p = 0.04) and egg sensitization (9 vs. 15%; p = 0.02). This study highlights that fish oil supplementation during the second half of the pregnancy may provide an effective strategy to reduce the risk of eczema and food sensitization.

In another study by the same group [73], 420 high-risk infants were randomized to DHA 280 mg plus EPA 110 mg daily, or olive oil (control) from birth to 6 months of age. Between-group comparisons revealed no differences in allergic sensitization, eczema, asthma or food allergy. While postnatal fish oil supplementation improved infant ω-3 fatty acid status, it did not prevent childhood allergic disease. This finding is in keeping with an earlier Swedish study that failed to find a preventive effect of postnatal omega-3 or omega-6 fatty acid exposure on eczema, asthma or atopic disease [74]. In summary, fish oil supplementation during pregnancy reduced the risk of atopic eczema and food sensitization, whereas dietary fish oil supplementation of the infant after birth was ineffective.

Vitamin D
Vitamin D is thought to be an important modulator of allergy risk in young infants [75, 76]. A recent Australian study showed that vitamin D insufficiency (serum level <50 nmol/l) was associated with a significantly increased risk of egg and/or peanut allergy [77]. This finding concurred with the observation that the prevalence of food allergy and eczema follows a North-South gradient, being more common in regions with less sun exposure and lower skin-derived vitamin D levels [78]. Adequate vitamin D levels in the first year of life may therefore provide protection against the development of food allergies. By contrast, vitamin D may also have undesirable immune-modulating effects and, in high doses, increase the risk of allergic sensitization. Vitamin D has been shown to inhibit the maturation of dendritic cells and impede the development of T helper 1 responses. In theory, vitamin D therefore could increase the risk of allergic disorders in infancy [79]. This is supported by a recent German birth cohort study (LINA study) which found that high vitamin D levels during pregnancy and at birth were associated with an increased risk of food allergy [80]. The varying effects of vitamin D on allergy risk have been explained by a U-shaped dose-response curve, whereby normal vitamin D levels may confer a protective effect and higher levels may increase the allergy risk [76]. The aforementioned studies suggest that both vitamin D insufficiency and oversupplementation are risk factors for allergies [75]. A well-designed, prospective randomized trial is needed to assess the role and optimum dosage of vitamin D supplementation in pregnant women and young infants.

Conclusions

Tolerance development and allergy risk are influenced by a complex array of factors, including genetics, epigenetic imprinting, microbial environment and other environmental factors. Strategies to promote early gut colonization with diverse, bifidobacteria-rich fecal microbiota include breastfeeding, avoidance of surgical deliveries or of perinatal antibiotics (where possible), and living in a rural farm environment. Exclusive breastfeeding for 6 months, use of hydrolyzed formula when breastfeeding is not possible, and the delayed introduction of complementary feeding from 4 to 6 months remain the main strategies in primary prevention of dietary allergy. Several studies have demonstrated a beneficial effect of probiotics, particularly in the prevention of atopic dermatitis. The role of prebiotics in food allergy prevention is at this stage less clear. LC-PUFA supplementation (fish oil, DHA, EPA) during pregnancy has been shown to stimulate regulatory T cell responses and may reduce the risk of atopic dermatitis and egg sensitization. Fish oil supplementation in the newborn had no preventive effect for later allergic disease. The role of vitamin D supplementation during pregnancy and early infancy for the purpose of allergy prevention requires further study.

Disclosure Statement

Dr. Heine is a member of the Scientific Advisory Boards of the Nestlé Nutrition Institute (Oceania) and Nutricia/Danone (Australia). He has participated in industry-funded education activities.

References

1 Sicherer SH: Epidemiology of food allergy. J Allergy Clin Immunol 2011;127:594–602.
2 Ho MH, Lee SL, Wong WH, et al: Prevalence of self-reported food allergy in Hong Kong children and teens – a population survey. Asian Pac J Allergy Immunol 2012;30:275–284.
3 Shek LP, Cabrera-Morales EA, Soh SE, et al: A population-based questionnaire survey on the prevalence of peanut, tree nut, and shellfish allergy in 2 Asian populations. J Allergy Clin Immunol 2010;126:324–331, 331 e1–7.
4 Mullins RJ: Paediatric food allergy trends in a community-based specialist allergy practice, 1995–2006. Med J Aust 2007;186:618–621.
5 Osborne NJ, Koplin JJ, Martin PE, et al, Health Nuts Investigators: Prevalence of challenge-proven IgE-mediated food allergy using population-based sampling and predetermined challenge criteria in infants. J Allergy Clin Immunol 2011;127:668–676 e1–2.
6 van den Oord RA, Sheikh A: Filaggrin gene defects and risk of developing allergic sensitisation and allergic disorders: systematic review and meta-analysis. BMJ 2009;339:b2433.
7 Liu M, Rogers L, Cheng Q, et al: Genetic variants of TSLP and asthma in an admixed urban population. PLoS One 2011;6:e25099.
8 Sherrill JD, Gao PS, Stucke EM, et al: Variants of thymic stromal lymphopoietin and its receptor associate with eosinophilic esophagitis. J Allergy Clin Immunol 2010;126:160–165 e3.
9 Martino DJ, Prescott SL: Progress in understanding the epigenetic basis for immune development, immune function, and the rising incidence of allergic disease. Curr Allergy Asthma Rep 2013;13:85–92.
10 Michel S, Busato F, Genuneit J, et al, PASTURE Study Group: Farm exposure and time trends in early childhood may influence DNA methylation in genes related to asthma and allergy. Allergy 2013;68:355–364.
11 Prescott SL: Effects of early cigarette smoke exposure on early immune development and respiratory disease. Paediatr Respir Rev 2008; 9:3–9, quiz 10.
12 Johnson CL, Versalovic J: The human microbiome and its potential importance to pediatrics. Pediatrics 2012;129:950–960.
13 Palmer C, Bik EM, DiGiulio DB, et al: Development of the human infant intestinal microbiota. PLoS Biol 2007;5:e177.

14 Lopez P, Gonzalez-Rodríguez I, Sanchez B, et al: Interaction of *Bifidobacterium bifidum* LMG13195 with HT29 cells influences regulatory-T-cell-associated chemokine receptor expression. Appl Environ Microbiol 2012;78:2850–2857.

15 Isolauri E: Development of healthy gut microbiota early in life. J Paediatr Child Health 2012;48(suppl 3):1–6.

16 Dominguez-Bello MG, Costello EK, Contreras M, et al: Delivery mode shapes the acquisition and structure of the initial microbiota across multiple body habitats in newborns. Proc Natl Acad Sci USA 2010;107:11971–11975.

17 Thavagnanam S, Fleming J, Bromley A, et al: A meta-analysis of the association between Caesarean section and childhood asthma. Clin Exp Allergy 2008;38:629–633.

18 van Nimwegen FA, Penders J, Stobberingh EE, et al: Mode and place of delivery, gastrointestinal microbiota, and their influence on asthma and atopy. J Allergy Clin Immunol 2011;128:948–955 e1–3.

19 Penders J, Thijs C, van den Brandt PA, et al: Gut microbiota composition and development of atopic manifestations in infancy: the KOALA Birth Cohort Study. Gut 2007;56:661–667.

20 Riedler J, Eder W, Oberfeld G, Schreuer M: Austrian children living on a farm have less hay fever, asthma and allergic sensitization. Clin Exp Allergy 2000;30:194–200.

21 Ege MJ: Intestinal microbial diversity in infancy and allergy risk at school age. J Allergy Clin Immunol 2011;128:653–654.

22 Ege MJ, Mayer M, Normand AC, et al, GABRIELA Transregio 22 Study Group: Exposure to environmental microorganisms and childhood asthma. N Engl J Med 2011;364:701–709.

23 Abrahamsson TR, Jakobsson HE, Andersson AF, et al: Low diversity of the gut microbiota in infants with atopic eczema. J Allergy Clin Immunol 2012;129:434–440, 440 e1–2.

24 Ismail IH, Oppedisano F, Joseph SJ, et al: Reduced gut microbial diversity in early life is associated with later development of eczema but not atopy in high-risk infants. Pediatr Allergy Immunol 2012;23:674–681.

25 Abrahamsson TR, Jakobsson T, Böttcher MF, et al: Probiotics in prevention of IgE-associated eczema: a double-blind, randomized, placebo-controlled trial. J Allergy Clin Immunol 2007;119:1174–1180.

26 Kukkonen K, Savilahti E, Haahtela T, et al: Probiotics and prebiotic galacto-oligosaccharides in the prevention of allergic diseases: a randomized, double-blind, placebo-controlled trial. J Allergy Clin Immunol 2007;119:192–198.

27 Kramer MS: Breastfeeding and allergy: the evidence. Ann Nutr Metab 2011;59(suppl 1):20–26.

28 Greer FR, Sicherer SH, Burks AW, American Academy of Pediatrics Committee on Nutrition, American Academy of Pediatrics Section on Allergy and Immunology: Effects of early nutritional interventions on the development of atopic disease in infants and children: the role of maternal dietary restriction, breastfeeding, timing of introduction of complementary foods, and hydrolyzed formulas. Pediatrics 2008;121:183–191.

29 ESPGHAN Committee on Nutrition, Agostoni C, Decsi T, Fewtrell M, et al: Complementary feeding: a commentary by the ESPGHAN Committee on Nutrition. J Pediatr Gastroenterol Nutr 2008;46:99–110.

30 Prescott SL, Tang ML, Australasian Society of Clinical Immunology and Allergy: The Australasian Society of Clinical Immunology and Allergy position statement: summary of allergy prevention in children. Med J Aust 2005;182:464–467.

31 Kramer MS, Matush L, Vanilovich I, et al: Promotion of Breastfeeding Intervention Trial Study Group: Effect of prolonged and exclusive breast feeding on risk of allergy and asthma: cluster randomised trial. BMJ 2007;335:815.

32 Grzeskowiak L, Collado MC, Mangani C, et al: Distinct gut microbiota in southeastern African and northern European infants. J Pediatr Gastroenterol Nutr 2012;54:812–816.

33 Saarinen UM, Kajosaari M: Breastfeeding as prophylaxis against atopic disease: prospective follow-up study until 17 years old. Lancet 1995;346:1065–1069.

34 Gdalevich M, Mimouni D, David M, Mimouni M: Breast-feeding and the onset of atopic dermatitis in childhood: a systematic review and meta-analysis of prospective studies. J Am Acad Dermatol 2001;45:520–527.

35 Snijders BE, Thijs C, Dagnelie PC, et al: Breast-feeding duration and infant atopic manifestations, by maternal allergic status, in the first 2 years of life (KOALA study). J Pediatr 2007;151:347–351, 351 e1–2.

36 Mihrshahi S, Ampon R, Webb K, et al, CAPS Team: The association between infant feeding practices and subsequent atopy among children with a family history of asthma. Clin Exp Allergy 2007;37:671–679.

37 Matheson MC, Erbas B, Balasuriya A, et al: Breast-feeding and atopic disease: a cohort study from childhood to middle age. J Allergy Clin Immunol 2007;120:1051–1057.

38 Osborn DA, Sinn J: Formulas containing hydrolysed protein for prevention of allergy and food intolerance in infants. Cochrane Database Syst Rev 2006:CD003664.

39 von Berg A, Koletzko S, Grubl A, et al, German Infant Nutritional Intervention Study Group: The effect of hydrolyzed cow's milk formula for allergy prevention in the first year of life: the German Infant Nutritional Intervention Study, a randomized double-blind trial. J Allergy Clin Immunol 2003;111:533–540.

40 Lowe AJ, Hosking CS, Bennett CM, et al: Effect of a partially hydrolyzed whey infant formula at weaning on risk of allergic disease in high-risk children: a randomized controlled trial. J Allergy Clin Immunol 2011;128:360–365 e4.

41 Alexander DD, Cabana MD: Partially hydrolyzed 100% whey protein infant formula and reduced risk of atopic dermatitis: a meta-analysis. J Pediatr Gastroenterol Nutr 2010; 50:422–430.

42 Su J, Prescott S, Sinn J, et al: Cost-effectiveness of partially-hydrolyzed formula for prevention of atopic dermatitis in Australia. J Med Econ 2012;15:1064–1077.

43 Iskedjian M, Dupont C, Spieldenner J, et al: Economic evaluation of a 100% whey-based, partially hydrolysed formula in the prevention of atopic dermatitis among French children. Curr Med Res Opin 2010;26:2607–2626.

44 Iskedjian M, Belli D, Farah B, et al: Economic evaluation of a 100% whey-based partially hydrolyzed infant formula in the prevention of atopic dermatitis among Swiss children. J Med Econ 2012;15:378–393.

45 Lowe AJ, Dharmage SC, Allen KJ, et al: The role of partially hydrolyzed whey formula for the prevention of allergic disease: evidence and gaps. Expert Rev Clin Immunol 2013;9:31–41.

46 ESPGHAN Committee on Nutrition, Agostoni C, Axelsson I, Goulet O, et al: Soy protein infant formulae and follow-on formulae: a commentary by the ESPGHAN Committee on Nutrition. J Pediatr Gastroenterol Nutr 2006;42:352–361.

47 Osborn DA, Sinn J: Soy formula for prevention of allergy and food intolerance in infants. Cochrane Database Syst Rev 2006:CD003741.

48 Turck D: Soy protein for infant feeding: what do we know? Curr Opin Clin Nutr Metab Care 2007;10:360–365.

49 Hill DJ, Murch SH, Rafferty K, et al: The efficacy of amino acid-based formulas in relieving the symptoms of cow's milk allergy: a systematic review. Clin Exp Allergy 2007;37:808–822.

50 Chehade M, Mayer L: Oral tolerance and its relation to food hypersensitivities. J Allergy Clin Immunol 2005;115:3–12, quiz 13.

51 Fergusson DM, Horwood LJ, Shannon FT: Early solid feeding and recurrent childhood eczema: a 10-year longitudinal study. Pediatrics 1990;86:541–546.

52 Filipiak B, Zutavern A, Koletzko S, et al, GINI Group: Solid food introduction in relation to eczema: results from a four-year prospective birth cohort study. J Pediatr 2007; 151:352–358.

53 Fiocchi A, Assa'ad A, Bahna S, Adverse Reactions to Foods Committee, American College of Allergy, Asthma and Immunology: Food allergy and the introduction of solid foods to infants: a consensus document. Adverse Reactions to Foods Committee, American College of Allergy, Asthma and Immunology. Ann Allergy Asthma Immunol 2006;97:10–20, quiz 21, 77.

54 Prescott SL, Smith P, Tang M, et al: The importance of early complementary feeding in the development of oral tolerance: concerns and controversies. Pediatr Allergy Immunol 2008;19:375–380.

55 Palmer DJ, Makrides M: Diet of lactating women and allergic reactions in their infants. Curr Opin Clin Nutr Metab Care 2006;9: 284–288.

56 Arshad SH, Bateman B, Sadeghnejad A, et al: Prevention of allergic disease during childhood by allergen avoidance: the Isle of Wight prevention study. J Allergy Clin Immunol 2007;119:307–313.

57 Kramer MS, Kakuma R: Maternal dietary antigen avoidance during pregnancy or lactation, or both, for preventing or treating atopic disease in the child. Cochrane Database Syst Rev 2012:CD000133.

58 Björkstén B: The epidemiology of food allergy. Curr Opin Allergy Clin Immunol 2001;1: 225–227.

59   Rautava S, Collado MC, Salminen S, Isolauri E: Probiotics modulate host-microbe interaction in the placenta and fetal gut: a randomized, double-blind, placebo-controlled trial. Neonatology 2012;102:178–184.

60   Kalliomäki M, Salminen S, Arvilommi H, et al: Probiotics in primary prevention of atopic disease: a randomised placebo-controlled trial. Lancet 2001;357:1076–1079.

61   Taylor AL, Dunstan JA, Prescott SL: Probiotic supplementation for the first 6 months of life fails to reduce the risk of atopic dermatitis and increases the risk of allergen sensitization in high-risk children: a randomized controlled trial. J Allergy Clin Immunol 2007; 119:184–191.

62   Fiocchi A, Burks W, Bahna SL, et al, The WAO Special Committee on Food Allergy and Nutrition: Clinical Use of Probiotics in Pediatric Allergy (CUPPA): A World Allergy Organization Position Paper. World Allergy Organ J 2012;5:148–167.

63   Donovan SM, Wang M, Li M, et al: Host-microbe interactions in the neonatal intestine: role of human milk oligosaccharides. Adv Nutr 2012;3:450S–455S.

64   Haarman M, Knol J: Quantitative real-time PCR analysis of fecal *Lactobacillus* species in infants receiving a prebiotic infant formula. Appl Environ Microbiol 2006;72:2359–2365.

65   Scholtens PA, Alles MS, Bindels JG, et al: Bifidogenic effects of solid weaning foods with added prebiotic oligosaccharides: a randomised controlled clinical trial. J Pediatr Gastroenterol Nutr 2006;42:553–559.

66   Moro G, Arslanoglu S, Stahl B, et al: A mixture of prebiotic oligosaccharides reduces the incidence of atopic dermatitis during the first six months of age. Arch Dis Child 2006;91: 814–819.

67   Grüber C, van Stuijvenberg M, Mosca F, et al, MIPS-1 Working Group: Reduced occurrence of early atopic dermatitis because of immunoactive prebiotics among low-atopy-risk infants. J Allergy Clin Immunol 2010; 126:791–797.

68   Osborn DA, Sinn JK: Prebiotics in infants for prevention of allergic disease and food hypersensitivity. Cochrane Database Syst Rev 2007:CD006474.

69   Prescott SL, Dunstan JA: Prenatal fatty acid status and immune development: the pathways and the evidence. Lipids 2007;42:801–810.

70   Dunstan JA, Mitoulas LR, Dixon G, et al: The effects of fish oil supplementation in pregnancy on breast milk fatty acid composition over the course of lactation: a randomized controlled trial. Pediatr Res 2007;62:689–694.

71   Krauss-Etschmann S, Hartl D, Rzehak P, et al, Nutraceuticals for Healthier Life Study Group: Decreased cord blood IL-4, IL-13, and CCR4 and increased TGF-beta levels after fish oil supplementation of pregnant women. J Allergy Clin Immunol 2008;121: 464–470 e6.

72   Palmer DJ, Sullivan T, Gold MS, et al: Effect of n-3 long chain polyunsaturated fatty acid supplementation in pregnancy on infants' allergies in first year of life: randomised controlled trial. BMJ 2012;344:e184.

73   D'Vaz N, Meldrum SJ, Dunstan JA, et al: Postnatal fish oil supplementation in high-risk infants to prevent allergy: randomized controlled trial. Pediatrics 2012;130:674–682.

74   Almqvist C, Garden F, Xuan W, et al, CAPS Team: Omega-3 and omega-6 fatty acid exposure from early life does not affect atopy and asthma at age 5 years. J Allergy Clin Immunol 2007;119:1438–1444.

75   Paxton GA, Teale GR, Nowson CA, et al: Vitamin D and health in pregnancy, infants, children and adolescents in Australia and New Zealand: a position statement. Med J Aust 2013;198:142–143.

76   Wjst M: Is vitamin D supplementation responsible for the allergy pandemic? Curr Opin Allergy Clin Immunol 2012;12:257–262.

77   Allen KJ, Koplin JJ, Ponsonby AL, et al: Vitamin D insufficiency is associated with challenge-proven food allergy in infants. J Allergy Clin Immunol 2013;131:1109–1116, 1116. e1–6.

78   Osborne NJ, Ukoumunne OC, Wake M, Allen KJ: Prevalence of eczema and food allergy is associated with latitude in Australia. J Allergy Clin Immunol 2012;129:865–867.

79   Wjst M: The vitamin D slant on allergy. Pediatr Allergy Immunol 2006;17:477–483.

80   Weisse K, Winkler S, Hirche F, et al: Maternal and newborn vitamin D status and its impact on food allergy development in the German LINA cohort study. Allergy 2013;68: 220–228.

Black RE, Singhal A, Uauy R (eds): International Nutrition: Achieving Millennium Goals and Beyond.
Nestlé Nutr Inst Workshop Ser, vol 78, pp 155–160, (DOI: 10.1159/000354957)
Nestec Ltd., Vevey/S. Karger AG., Basel, © 2014

Nutrition and Chronic Disease: Lessons from the Developing and Developed World

Andrew M. Prentice

MRC International Nutrition Group, London School of Hygiene & Tropical Medicine, London, UK, and MRC Keneba, Keneba, The Gambia

Abstract

Many features of human susceptibility to chronic noncommunicable diseases can be mapped onto the framework of the match/mismatch hypothesis. From an evolutionary perspective, it is highly likely that the human genome has been under selective pressure to survive and reproduce against a background of seasonal food shortages and frequent episodic famines, leading to the attractive, but unproven, concept of 'a thrifty genotype made deleterious by famine'. From an ontogeny perspective, it has been clearly demonstrated that fetal undernutrition leads to a thrifty phenotype that enhances metabolic risk if the individual is later exposed to an energy-abundant environment. Data from developing and rapidly emerging countries permit insights into both of these pathways. Many populations are rapidly emerging from conditions broadly representative of human history over the past 600 or so generations (i.e. since the dawn of agriculture) and are transitioning within very few generations to a state of dietary abundance and low physical activity. And within this framework, many individuals make an even more rapid personal transition from the womb of a malnourished mother to a state of affluence. These journeys provide exceptional opportunities to interrogate thrifty genotype/phenotype theories, but such prospects are frequently impaired by a lack of robust data.

© 2014 Nestec Ltd., Vevey/S. Karger AG, Basel

Introduction

In a preceding chapter, Uauy et al. [pp. 39–52] have made the case that the very rapid demographic and nutrition transition affecting many emergent countries is precipitating a 'double burden' of disease. This double burden – the unfin-

Table 1. International Diabetes Federation projections for diabetes prevalence rates by 2030

Top 10: countries/territories of number (millions) of people with diabetes (20–79 years), 2011 and 2030

Country/territory	2011	Country/territory	2030
1. China	90.0	1. China	129.7
2. India	61.3	2. India	101.2
3. United States of America	23.7	3. United States of America	29.6
4. Russian Federation	12.6	4. Brazil	19.6
5. Brazil	12.4	5. Bangladesh	16.8
6. Japan	10.7	6. Mexico	16.4
7. Mexico	10.3	7. Russian Federation	14.1
8. Bangladesh	8.4	8. Egypt	12.4
9. Egypt	7.3	9. Indonesia	11.8
10. Indonesia	7.3	10. Pakistan	11.4

ished agenda of infectious diseases and the emergent agenda of chronic diseases – is a major threat to the development of nations.

The fact that developed nations have previously travelled down this road of abundant, low-cost, highly-refined, energy-dense diets combined with sedentary lifestyles, leading to fat gain and its associated morbidities, should hold lessons that could be used to slow the growing pandemic of noncommunicable diseases (NCDs). Conversely, knowledge gleaned from studying the rapid dynamics of change in developing countries may help to us to understand causal pathways with potentially important lessons for affluent societies. What are these lessons, and can we learn them fast enough to have a meaningful impact on global public health?

Diabetes: The Leading Exemplar of Double Burden Diseases

Among the wide range of chronic NCDs that hold a threat for emergent nations, diabetes stands out as the one that is most intimately linked to the societal changes that are transforming the disease landscape as countries pass through the nutrition and demographic transitions. Projections for the global increase in type 2 diabetes mellitus (T2D) leading up to 2030 are listed in table 1 which shows that, with the exception of the US, the countries with the leading burden will be those that are only now passing through the demographic transition. There are two synergistic components driving this change: first, the increases in child survival and adult longevity that allow longer exposure to any detrimental lifestyle factors, and, second, the rapid development of obesity.

It is well-proven that unhealthy weight gain lies on the causal pathway to metabolic syndrome, impaired glucose tolerance and ultimately to T2D. It is also clear that certain populations (e.g. South Asians, Polynesian Islanders, Pima Indians) are at a higher risk than others [Misra and Bhardwaj, this vol., pp. 133–140]. In the Pima Indians and Polynesians, much of this increased risk is mediated through their very high rates of early-onset obesity [1]. In South Asians, there is good evidence that they are more prone to obesity-related pathology at a lower body mass index (BMI) due to a relative excess of intra-abdominal adipose tissue [Misra and Bhardwaj, this vol., pp. 133–140]. Thus, BMI cutoffs are set at a lower level for South Indians [2].

The dyad of obesity and diabetes (sometimes termed 'diabesity') will be used as the key exemplar below, but the arguments are equally applicable to a range of other chronic diseases such as hypertension.

Exploiting Genetic Differences to Map Causal Pathways in Chronic Diseases

A question that arises from these observations is whether the differences summarized above are due to genotypic differences or life-course (including intergenerational) phenotypic differences, or a combination of the two. The issue of genetic variation clearly needs to be addressed when drawing comparisons between nations. The putative existence of 'thrifty genes' [3] is frequently invoked to explain the rapid transition towards obesity in urban Africans and South Asians, yet some of the known obesity-predisposing gene variants are less common in these populations. Intriguingly, for the human fat mass and obesity-associated (FTO) gene, which is the strongest of the known obesity-associated gene variants, the more recent variant allele favors leanness, not weight gain [4].

It is also a misconception to suggest that areas associated with recent famines and food-shortages (i.e. Africa and the Indian subcontinent) would have been under greater pressure to select thrifty genes. Historically, all populations worldwide have been under gene selection driven by famine [3], and the majority of this selection has probably been mediated through traits that influence fertility and reproductive success under marginal nutritional conditions [5]. Any such favorable genotypes may contribute to obesity, by favoring deposition of reproductively useful fat reserves in times of plenty [3], and to T2D, by favoring peripheral insulin resistance to benefit conception at low levels of BMI [5], and by displacing resources towards the fetus.

We [e.g. 3, 5, 6] and others [e.g. 7, 8] have written extensively about the possible role of thrifty genes in determining risk of obesity and T2D and speculated that definitive proof would shortly be available. However, the wait may need to continue as, although both traits are highly heritable, and large-scale genome-wide association studies (GWAS) have found multiple highly significant associations, even the most persuasive of these (i.e. FTO) has a very small influence on BMI, and when summed together all of the GWAS hits can still only explain a very small proportion of the heritability. New approaches involving integration of ENCODE analysis, systems biology approaches to genome-phenome analysis, and the analysis of genome-epigenome interactions may all yield future dividends. In the meantime, it will be more profitable to concentrate on potentially modifiable influences on chronic diseases.

Exploiting Phenotypic Differences to Map Causal Pathways in Chronic Diseases

The wide diversity of disease phenotypes (i.e. subvariants of insulin resistance/diabetes and hypertension), especially in populations of African origin, may be particularly helpful in efforts to map pathways of disease causality through GWAS and phenome-wide association studies. Recognition of this fact has resulted in increased investment in building cohorts and genetic repositories from such populations (e.g. H3A and the African Partnership for Chronic Disease Research) and will ultimately pay dividends in both developed and less developed populations.

Exploiting Rapid Development to Study Life-Course and Intergenerational Influences on Chronic Diseases

The basic thesis encapsulated in the developmental origins of adult disease (DOHAD) hypothesis is now generally well accepted [Singhal, this vol., pp. 123–132; Adair, this vol., pp. 111–120], but there remains much to be learnt about the mechanisms by which early life exposures affect chronic disease outcomes. The compression of the timeframe in which emerging societies are being exposed to affluent diets and lifestyles offers special opportunities to interrogate these mechanisms further, and considerable research is in progress concerning the long-term effects of nutritional deficits and excess as an individual passes through the various phases of the nutrient supply chain (histiotrophic, placental, mammary, weaning and through to adult diet). Matriline (and possibly patriline) influences on the capacity of such processes offer the opportunity for intergenerational effects on chronic disease outcomes, and these are also easier to study in rapidly transitioning societies, but with lessons applicable globally.

Exploiting the Nutritional Deprivations of Underdeveloped Societies to Understand Epigenetic Regulation of Disease

Epigenetic variations are currently viewed as likely mediators of the known associations between early-life nutritional exposures and later disease – the DOHAD thesis. This topic represents another good example of where research in rapidly developing nations can have global implications. Some of the first proof-of-principle studies in humans are demonstrating that alterations in nutrients involved in maternal methyl-donor supply (choline, betaine, methionine, folate, vitamins B_2, B_6 and B_{12}) do affect methylation patterns of the offspring [9–11]. Such studies are often more tractable in populations with naturally low intake levels. The phenotypic and health implications of these changes are far from being understood, but a key emergent message is that different dietary practices can lead to a range of imbalances in methyl-donor metabolic cycles and that there will not be a single solution to optimizing such diets. For instance, B_{12} deficiency (especially against a background of folate repletion) appears to be a major issue in rural Indians [12] but not in rural Africans [13].

Future Prospects

The ultimate aim of all such research is to inform public health interventions that can reduce the penetrance of chronic diseases for future generations. Whether such interventions can be effective against the inherent propensity for gluttony and sloth in human populations remains to be seen.

Disclosure Statement

The author has no conflicts of interest.

References

1 King H, Zimmet P: Trends in the prevalence and incidence of diabetes: non-insulin-dependent diabetes mellitus. World Health Stat Q 1988;41:190–196.

2 WHO Expert Consultation: Appropriate body-mass index for Asian populations and its implications for policy and intervention strategies. Lancet 2004;363:157–163.

3 Prentice AM: Early influences on human energy regulation: thrifty genotypes and thrifty phenotypes. Physiol Behav 2005;86:640–652.

4 Frayling TM, Ong K: Piecing together the FTO jigsaw. Genome Biol 2011;12:104.

5 Corbett SJ, McMichael AJ, Prentice AM: Type 2 diabetes, cardiovascular disease, and the evolutionary paradox of the polycystic ovary syndrome: a fertility first hypothesis. Am J Hum Biol 2009;21:587–598.

6 Prentice AM, Hennig BJ, Fulford AJ: Evolutionary origins of the obesity epidemic: natural selection of thrifty genes or genetic drift following predation release? Int J Obes (Lond) 2008;32:1607–1610.

7 Diamond J: The double puzzle of diabetes. Nature 2003;423:599–602.

8 Joffe B, Zimmet P: The thrifty genotype in type 2 diabetes: an unfinished symphony moving to its finale? Endocrine 1998;9:139–141.

9 Khulan B, Cooper WN, Skinner BM, et al: Periconceptional maternal micronutrient supplementation is associated with widespread gender related changes in the epigenome: a study of a unique resource in the Gambia. Hum Mol Genet 2012;21:2086–2101.

10 Cooper WN, Khulan B, Owens S, et al: DNA methylation profiling at imprinted loci after periconceptional micronutrient supplementation in humans: results of a pilot randomized controlled trial. FASEB J 2012;26:1782–1790.

11 Waterland RA, Kellermayer R, Laritsky E, et al: Season of conception in rural Gambia affects DNA methylation at putative human metastable epialleles. PLoS Genet 2010; 6:e1001252.

12 Yajnik CS, Deshpande SS, Jackson AA, et al: Vitamin B12 and folate concentrations during pregnancy and insulin resistance in the offspring: the Pune Maternal Nutrition Study. Diabetologia 2008;51:29–38.

13 Dominguez-Salas P, Moore SE, Cole D, et al: DNA methylation potential: dietary intake and blood concentrations of one-carbon metabolites and cofactors in rural African women. Am J Clin Nutr 2013;97:1217–1227.

Black RE, Singhal A, Uauy R (eds): International Nutrition: Achieving Millennium Goals and Beyond.
Nestlé Nutr Inst Workshop Ser, vol 78, pp 161–162, (DOI: 10.1159/000354961)
Nestec Ltd., Vevey/S. Karger AG., Basel, © 2014

Summary on Future Perspectives

The final section of the workshop took a different tack to the previous two sessions. Rather than focusing on meeting Millennium Development Goals, this section highlighted the health impact of noncommunicable disease in both richer and poorer nations. *Atul Singhal* set the scene by reviewing the global disease burden associated with noncommunicable disease and in particular mortality from cardiovascular disease, 80% of which occurs in low- or middle-income countries. His presentation emphasized the importance of early-life feeding practices such as breastfeeding, optimizing the patterns of infant growth, and preventing early addition of complementary feeding in helping to prevent later obesity and atherosclerotic cardiovascular disease. Evidence was presented to support the role of early-life nutrition from both developed and developing countries and on potential mechanisms such as the role of infant growth/nutrition in affecting appetite regulation. The risk-benefit of slower weight gain in infancy on later health was a particular focus of subsequent group discussions. Whilst there is substantial evidence that too fast infant weight gain from a high nutrient intake in infancy could increase the risk of later obesity and cardiovascular disease (without benefit to other health outcomes), whether these data applied to middle- and low-income countries was uncertain. Therefore, a 'one size fits all' policy for infant nutrition was unlikely to be ideal.

Anoop Misra eloquently continued the theme of noncommunicable disease in developing countries, focusing on the rapid increase in obesity and type 2 diabetes, particularly in children and in South Asian populations. Alarmingly, he highlighted the fact that a third of the urban population in India had the metabolic syndrome mainly as the result of increased consumption of energy-dense 'fast foods' and a sedentary lifestyle. South Asians were at particular risk of insulin resistance and the metabolic syndrome because of higher percentage fat relative to BMI when compared to Whites, more intra-abdominal or visceral adiposity, and more fat deposition in ectopic sites such as skeletal muscles and the liver. As a consequence, *Anoop Misra* emphasized that optimizing lifestyle was critical in South Asians, starting from intrauterine nutrition but continuing throughout childhood into adult life.

The importance of early-life feeding practices for the prevention of chronic disease was also emphasized by *Ralf Heine*, but this time for food allergies and atopic diseases. A theme common to the prevention of obesity and cardiovascular disease as well as allergic disease was the importance of breastfeeding for the first 6 months, and the introduction of solids between 4 and 6 months. Potential mechanisms for the benefits of breastfeeding were reviewed and included the effects on the gut microbiome in modulating immune regulation and tolerance. For infants not breastfed, perinatal supplementation with prebiotics and/or probiotics was shown to reduce the risk of atopic dermatitis, but not food allergy or respiratory allergies. *Ralf Heine* also discussed potentially newer therapies for prevention of atopic disease including the role of vitamin D deficiency (or excess) and maternal fish oil supplementation. His comprehensive review was greatly appreciated and stimulated much discussion particularly on the scientific mechanisms and the clinical implications of different early nutritional interventions for the prevention of atopic disease.

The final presentation was given by *Andrew Prentice*. In a highly stimulating and challenging insight, he gave an overview of lessons that could be learnt from developed countries to slow the global pandemic of noncommunicable diseases, while lessons from developing countries undergoing rapid changes were helping our understanding of causal pathways. He chose obesity/type 2 diabetes as the leading example of a 'double burden' disease and highlighted the extensive evidence from richer countries for the role of lifestyle factors in its development, while evidence from the developing world increased our understanding of the role of genetic factors in its etiology. For instance, surprisingly, gene variants predisposing to obesity were found to be less common than expected in some populations from developing countries at high risk of obesity and diabetes. *Andrew Prentice* reviewed the evidence for the role of 'thrifty genes' in the development of obesity/diabetes and the recent evidence in humans showing that maternal nutritional factors can lead to DNA methylation changes in the offspring. However, whether this knowledge will lead to interventions to prevent obesity and diabetes currently remains unknown.

Overall, the 'Future Perspectives' session of the workshop provided an excellent perspective on the problems facing the developing world in the next 20 years. The session produced much lively debate and clearly highlighted the importance of optimizing early nutrition for the prevention of the main health problems facing richer and poorer countries alike.

Atul Singhal

Subject Index

Demographic Health Survey (DHS) 30, 36
Diabetes, *see* Noncommunicable diseases
Disability-adjusted life years (DALYs), micronutrient deficiencies 24, 25
Dyslipidemia, *see* Noncommunicable diseases

Elimination diets, allergy prevention 146
Epigenetics
    developmental origins of disease 129
    Dutch famine adults 114, 115

Folic acid, pregnancy
    supplementation 88, 89
Food security 56, 60, 96, 97
Formula, allergy prevention
    amino acid-based formula 145
    hydrolyzed formula 144, 145
    soy formula 145
Fortification, foods 65

Human immunodeficiency virus
    (HIV) 44, 45
Hygiene hypothesis 142
Hypertension, *see* Noncommunicable diseases

India, obesity and metabolic syndrome
    community interventions 138
    overview 134–136
    prevention and control 136–138
INTERGROWTH study 50
Intrauterine growth restriction, *see* Small for gestational age
Iodine, deficiency 24
Iron deficiency
    anemia 24, 25
    pregnancy supplementation 74, 75, 77
    sweet potato consumption 101

Life course approach, nutrition 46, 47

Malnutrition, *see* Overnutrition; Undernutrition
Metabolic syndrome, *see also* Noncommunicable diseases
    South Asia

overview 134–136
    prevention and control 136–138
Millennium Development Goals (MDGs)
    13, 14, 55–57, 60, 67, 93–96, 102–105, 112, 117

Noncommunicable diseases (NCDs),
    see also Obesity
    complementary feeding studies 117, 128
    developmental origins 124, 125
    early postnatal factors 116, 117, 125, 126
    growth in cardiovascular disease
        programming
        infants 126–128
        children 128
    malnutrition double burden 40, 41
    mechanisms 129, 130
    overnutrition 45, 46
    overview 123, 124
    pregnancy studies 113–115
    public health implications of early nutrition 130
    small for gestational age 116
    undernutrition induction 45, 46

Obesity, *see also* Noncommunicable
    diseases; Overnutrition
    growth in cardiovascular disease
        programming
        infants 126–128
        children 128
    South Asia
        community interventions in India 138
        overview 134–136
        prevention and control 136–138
Omega-3 fatty acids, pregnancy
    supplementation 74, 75
Overnutrition, *see also* Obesity
    double burden of malnutrition 40–45, 47–49
    late effects 45, 46
    malnutrition operational definition 49–51
    mortality by risk factor and income 43